Dedication

To my husband, Corey, who believes in me, sometimes
more than I believe in myself—I love you so very
much. You have been my rock, my inspiration, and
my support. For all of these things, thank you.
To my children—Corey Jr., Kennedi and Aaliyah—
my love for you grows more and more each
an every day. You are my light and joy!
To my mom who has never left my side and
who encourages, loves and supports me through
everything—Thank you! You've made me better.

***

In remembrance of my dad, Howard "Bo" J. Gordon—
your love is never forgotten. I'll always be Daddy's Girl.
My great-grandmother, Mrs. Laura J. Cain,
your prayers were not in vain.

My brother Tyrone Gordon, I will continue
to make you proud. Thank you for your love,
guidance, and support. I love you so much.
My niece, Jamanda R. Gordon words will never be able
to express how much you mean to me. I love you!

***

A special acknowledgement and dedication of love to
Mrs. Yvette DeLane Wren-Collins. While I only had
you in my life briefly, your smile, your heart, and your
presence live on. Thank you for pouring into me while
fighting a battle of your own. I love you tremendously.

Acknowledgments

To my husband, Corey, and our children—Corey Jr., Kennedi, and Aaliyah—I would not have made it through this battle without you. You inspire me daily and keep me going.

To my mom, you are so amazing. Your strength and love give me direction, hope, and motivation.

To my best friends, Brandi Henry, and Zundra Bryant—I don't know what I would have done without you. Thank you for your love, time, and your heart.

To Drummond Bryant, thank you for your love, support, and for being there for all of us!

To my sisters and brothers—Jerry (Lucy), Howard, Tracy, Sharon, Jimmy, Tyrone (Robin), Ivory, Terry, Anothony—thank you for your love and support, for the meals, and the pies.

My sisters by choice—Nikki B., Kanisha, Tanesha, Lashonda and Sheena—you light up my life! I'm so blessed to have each of you. You are so amazing, and I'm thankful for your consistency, love, and the joy you've brought into my life.

Leticia Avery, you are forever in my heart! Thank you for just being you!

My cousins and first best friends, Chazsaty and Tacarra, I love you so much.

To all of my aunts and uncles that called and visited, thank you for your love, thoughts, and prayers.

Laura Marbs, Kris Maassen, Team Houston, and my entire ESI family—you guys rock! I appreciate your support, encouragement, and everything you've done to support my family during our journey.

Moma Barb K., I love you!

Tracee Green, you are one of a kind! I'm so grateful for you!

To the Pink Angels Foundation and Chantelle Nickson-Clark: Thank you for pouring into me, believing in me, and encouraging me throughout this journey. Thank you for your testimony and for being a great example of what being a survivor looks like. Thank you for helping me turn my pain into purpose.

To Maimah Karmo, founder and CEO of the Tigerlily Foundation, thank you for being fierce and amazing and for giving me the opportunity to advocate for my pink sisters! You inspire me to be better!

To all of my family and friends, co-workers, and church family, thank you for your support, prayers, and encouragement. I'm blessed to have a village as amazing as this!

To my amazing care team at SSM Health St. Peters and Lake St. Louis, Renaissance Plastic Surgeons—no thank you is big enough!

Dr. Aislinn Vaughan—Medical Director, Breast Surgeon, SSM Medical Group

ACKNOWLEDGMENTS

Dr. Pascale Salem—Hematology, Oncology, Internal Medicine, SSM Medical Group

Dr. Anna Fu—Radiation Oncology, SSM Medical Group

Dr. Paul Mills—Renaissance Plastic Surgery

Rebecca Florian—RN, CNOR Breast Health Specialist

Cancer Center Lake St. Louis Chemotherapy Nursing team, Cancer Center Kisker Road Radiology nurses and tech staff, SSM Emergency Room staff—*thank you for saving my life and being kind in the process.*

Prayer

Our Father who art in heaven, hallowed be thy name.
Thy kingdom come, thy will be done, on earth as it is in
heaven. Give us this day our daily bread. And forgive us
our trespasses as we forgive those who trespass against us.
And lead us not into temptation, but deliver us from evil.
Giving reverence to you, Father, as I write and you lead.
Let this book be what you've called it to be. I thank you
for all that has been done and all that will be done.
In Jesus's name. Amen.

Foreword

The Evolution of Me relates so clearly to the kinds of challenges cancer survivors face on a daily basis. The rawness and vulnerability Anastasia Stevenson shares will make just about anyone take a different outlook on life. We all face challenges and ups and downs, but to know that life can completely be turned upside down in a blink of an eye can be terrifying. It's not easy sharing the behind the scene parts that no one talks about; it takes courage. Anastasia knew that people in the world needed just that: Courage.

This book can be inspirational to others whether they are fighting challenges such as cancer or having everyday life challenges, for it demonstrates human resilience. It shows that we don't have to be victimized by ill health or hard times. Instead, we can use those seasons to build up our faith and pray more than ever before.

Anastasia provides a great example for others on how faith only grows stronger when it's tested. As you read through *The Evolution of Me*, I hope it encourages you as much as it encourages me to push through, even when times get hard. This is a story of hope, love, faith, and strength. Thank God that this woman overcame the incredible odds that she did in order to share with others around the world.

I have been honored to be in the presence of Anastasia and witness firsthand her determination to help others, even with what she was going through. I am amazed that going through this journey, Anastasia went one step further by birthing Evolution of Me LLC where she will continue to encourage and uplift other women along the way. Her determination and courage shine through in every word. This book is truly a detailed evolution of hope.

—Kanisha Anthony, Author, *Scarless—A Woman's Journey to Finding Her Strength and Identity*

Contents

Introduction

It was a beautiful Friday afternoon, but I had been holding my breath for the past few days. Today, in just a few minutes, I would receive *the* phone call.

"Hello, am I speaking with Anastasia Stevenson?"

I replied, "You are."

"Hi Anastasia, this is Dr. Vaughn. I wanted to call you as promised before the weekend with your results. I'm so sorry to let you know that the results came back, and they are positive for breast cancer in all three of the masses in your left breast."

Immediately, my mind began to wander. I still don't remember all of the details from that call. I just know I was happy to be on the passenger side instead of driving the car. It had been two weeks and three days since I discovered one lump in my left breast, and it was nothing but the Holy Spirit that nudged me to do my self-breast exam in the shower that Tuesday evening. I hadn't done it the month of January, and I'm certain I didn't do a good examination of myself in December.

Am I going to die? Is this my final chapter? were the immediate questions that came to mind after speaking with Dr. Vaughn.

And then I looked to my husband who answered that question without any hesitation. He said, "No matter what, we'll get through this together with God on our side." He had made the decision that I had not yet come around to. We were going to approach this as aggressively as the doctor recommended, and we'd be fine on the other side.

It took some time for me to come to that conclusion. I went through a period of denial, then anger, followed by sadness and frustration. I had overall been a fairly healthy person. No, I didn't eat the best, but I took care of myself. I didn't work out five days per week, but with three children, inclusive of a set of twin three-year-olds, I got my exercise. I didn't smoke and only had two or three glasses of wine a week, nothing excessive or what I would consider to be over the top. But here I was with a new diagnosis that would surely change life as I knew it.

I went through the fire and came out different and better. Through this process, there was an evolution. I evolved mentally, physically, spiritually, and emotionally. I learned that I am not in control and never have been. I learned that through one of the most difficult times of my life, I was strong, courageous, and built to stand the test of time. Evolution was a gift for the pain, and it allowed me to provide you a story of trial and triumph on love, family, business, and most importantly, self! Some might call it beauty for ashes.

Learning to love yourself in the fullness of who God has called you to be is a remarkable and gratifying feeling. To be lost in God's love for you through painful, uncomfortable, and difficult times produces diamonds—unbreakable and extremely valuable. In complete transparency through my encounter with breast cancer, I invite you to plug in your own story of trial. Any trial is able to produce and encourage an evolution of self-determination, goals, and daily inspirations; a trial that will bring about a desire for change, not living the same and a desire to be and want more; in fact, a desire to lean into the fullness and glory, abundance, and overflow that God himself created for you.

The flow of this book will consist of a Bible verse that inspires each chapter followed by the details. I've also included the journal entries that I kept via CaringBridge (an online resource to update friends and family during the breast cancer journey). This journal served as an outlet for me to pour out my feelings and thoughts and additionally allowed my friends and family to be a part of the progress. It also was a way to decrease the amount of times I needed to repeat information. I encourage you to also leverage journaling as you feel the need through this book to assess and address your potential opportunities. I prefer what I've called the GAP method. This is capturing Growth (from what is written), Acknowledgement (that this is an area you would like to evolve in), and a Prayer (for revelation knowledge and strength). Allow yourself to be vulnerable, and journey into your next evolution. And remember, there's always more than one.

Chapter 1

The Beginning

They who dwell in the ends of the earth stand in
awe of Your signs [the evidence of your presence].
You make the dawn and the sunset shout for joy.
—Psalms 65:8 (AMP)

To be in awe of God is an understatement. To understand his depth, strength, and power is to be forever in a state of wonder, amazement, and appreciation. As I begin this chapter, I am staring out of the window of a plane. I have on my right the glory of the clouds, the big never-ending clear blue sky, and a beautiful view of the sun, so bright and clear. As we proceed to my next destination, I once again peek out of the window and catch a glimpse of another 747-air flight traveling to a different destination but through the same clouds in the same beautiful sky…how amazing is that!

On the ground, these capsules are enormous, and in the eyes of a child, I can only imagine the stare of awe! But to see another in the air in passing is an incredible reflection of how God carries us through the known and unknown, through clear skies, dark clouds, and rain.

Travelling via the big blue sky has never been a *must do!* As a matter of fact, it for some is an "only if I have to" kind of thing. We forget that these luxuries, while very normal to us, are still a rather new concept. To allow yourself permission to let go and let God through words is an extremely easy thing to do, but in practice, it is much more difficult.

This brings me to the awe of God that I have as I travel through the mountains and valleys of breast cancer. As I grow, learn, and shift, I am becoming more aware of what my "must do" is and what I am able to determine and call a luxury. Living and not giving in to this disease is a must do. Conquering to tell the story and provide insight and inspiration is a must do. Giving encouragement and inspiration is a luxury. A great friend told me as I started on this journey that "this book is not for anyone else—it's for you and you alone. If it helps someone else, that's a God thing!" It's with those words in mind that I begin to write.

What I know about travelling is there is usually a reason in mind to leave one destination to get to another, whether it be a friend's wedding, vacation plans, an amazing girls' trip or a requirement for business. Unless you have an unlimited amount of time, you're going to choose the quickest and least painful way of getting there. For illustration purposes, that quick and painless way will be by plane. I mean, feel free to use the car, but in many ways, you're limiting yourself. You most certainly cannot travel by train, car, or bus from St. Louis, Missouri, to Paris, France (where I am now and one of my dream destinations)!

The same applies to embracing the calling on your life. God is with you. He has made the path. Though uncomfortable, inconvenient, and downright painful, all of your needs are supplied! Though you cannot see the signs to guide you to the next destination, you trust that the plane is carrying you in the right direction. You are a passenger. You don't need to know the details. Just sit, take in the peace, and enjoy the ride. Just on the other side of the clouds is the new destination to continue the growth, plan, and the path, becoming ready for the next.

My destination was evolution, and my method of travel was breast cancer. Every day, I am faced with choices. Choices to do, be, exist, impact, or change. I ask myself often, are these things from God? I don't want to do anything in vain. I look at women and men who have been, done, and overcome situations. They push me to want to do, be, exist, impact, and change myself and others that are around me. They push me to desire to serve and be of service. I choose this method to be the example, the vessel that God uses to do wonderful things. In this season of my life—without my choosing or permission—that vessel happens to be stage two (2) breast cancer.

> We shall walk by faith and not by
> sight. (2 Corinthians 5:7 KJV)

On the night of February 6, 2009, while taking a shower before bed, I heard a small voice that told me to do my routine self-breast exam. As with prior exams, I felt like this would be ordinary, nothing life-changing, just want I needed to do to be sure that I was healthy. What you should also know is that I have two daughters. Although they are young (only three years old), I have to practice what I preach, and what I will preach to them is that self-care is the best care.

This exam was different. I found a lump in my left breast. It was a small bump that I know hadn't been there in December when I last checked. The little bump immediately caused me to pause. I checked my right breast to compare and didn't feel anything. So I went back to my left breast to check again. I felt it again, and my stomach flopped. I was perplexed, and an overwhelming sense within me said, "Make a freaking appointment! At best it's nothing, a little something that needs to be checked, and we'll move on...but what if it's breast cancer?"

I finished my shower at a rapid pace and then got out. I picked up my cell phone and logged into my MyChart app and found the earliest appointment I could with my general physician. That appointment would be 11:00 a.m., Friday morning. Today was Wednesday the sixth—two days, no biggie! I continued my normal routine like any other day and made a brief mention to my husband, just saying I'd be working from home on Friday to go to a doctor's appointment for this thing I found, but no big deal. We proceeded as normal and went to bed. He assured me, as a good husband does, that everything would be fine, and he was sure it was nothing to worry about. I agreed... and then the next forty-eight hours seemed to drag on forever.

As I arrived at the doctor's office that Friday, February 8, I checked in and began to wait. I knew there needed to be a test or even a referral, so I stayed calm and went in for the breast exam. Alone in the room, I said a prayer: "God protect and prepare me for whatever this crap is or is not." Just that simple. Reflecting back on it, I'm speechless. I should have had support, someone to just talk to in the midst of all of this craziness, but I didn't know then what I would soon find out.

The doctor did her exam and confirmed there was something there. She said, "I want to get a closer look at it just to confirm. It could just be a little pocket of fluid, but it never hurts to just check it out."

I agreed, and off she went to write up my referral and have me meet with the scheduler to get it on the calendar sooner rather than later at the cancer center not too far from my home. The appointment was made for the following week. I had an ultrasound and a mammogram February 15. It was there that the technician confirmed I had not one but four masses across both breasts, three on the left and one on the right! *What in the entire hell did she just say?*

I had performed my breast exam and didn't feel anything else. She said, "As young as you are, your breast tissue is fairly dense, so it is completely understandable that you didn't feel those other masses."

Again, I went alone to this appointment...what was I thinking? Later on that day, Corey decided we needed a date day and a much-needed way to relieve some stress and be together, so we decided, like all couples, to go to the gun range! We took the kids to my mom to get some free time and release ourselves of responsibility for our babies to feel and say what we needed to feel and say without talking in code or waiting until they were asleep. It was a welcome release.

I shot a 9mm handgun, an assault rifle, and the mother of all machine guns! Funny thing is Corey had this idea—"What you see on the target you take out."—and the first thing that came to mind was breast cancer. With so much aggression, anger, and frustration, I hung the target, pushed it out, and grabbed the gun. All I could see were the words "breast cancer!" I shot like I had been shooting all my life. When we pulled the target back in, there were multiple holes right through the center of it. In my mind, I killed it, but there was still one thing—we hadn't received the call yet confirming that those masses were, in fact, breast cancer. Watch what you ask for and even how you frame your thoughts. I think I had resolved that this could, in fact, be breast cancer, but part of me was also still in denial that I was even in this place mentally and physically.

Another appointment was scheduled to have biopsies completed. The biopsies would take place on February 20 in the afternoon. This time, I knew I couldn't go alone, so my husband, Corey, and my mom accompanied me to this visit. I told my friend circles and my sisters and brothers to lift me in prayer as I had some appointments coming up that I needed extra support and prayer for. I didn't give any details but requested that I be added to the prayer list at church. They debated with me on telling them what was going on. However, I stood fast on the fact that once the appointments were over I would tell them everything they needed to know. Reality was, as far as family was concerned, only Corey, my mom, and I needed to know the intimate details of what was going on.

It felt that disclosing everything so soon when it could be nothing would be cruel punishment to those who loved me. Additionally, it was my decision on how I wanted to handle things, and this was what I could control. Reflecting and having conversations with them now, they weren't happy with my choice, but they understood the reasoning behind my decision.

I also decided to share this information with two other people who is strong pillars in my life—my boss at the time, Laura Marbs, and one of my mentors who happened to also be a two-time breast cancer survivor, Kris Maassen. I have always been transparent with Laura, and the longer I worked with her, the more she began to learn my mannerisms and could tell something was wrong. Laura also had a nursing background, and I could trust her to give me sound advice and encouragement as I prepared for the upcoming biopsy.

She was the first to let me know that I could and should give myself permission to be afraid! I had the tough girl mantra rocking. I kept a straight face and discussed it like I was giving instructions on how to make coffee, telling myself not to be fazed! This is what it was, or at least, that's what I wanted people to see. In reality, I wanted to go hide, wait, and just do nothing! She picked up on my feelings immediately. She looked me in my eyes and said, "You know this is not typical. It's not business, and you should not handle it that way. Give yourself permission to feel what you feel and know that it's okay, and I have your back no matter what!"

Immediately in her office, tears began to fall. I had found a person that I could truly be vulnerable with my full self and have no judgment brought against me. She promised to keep this between us, and it'd be my decision as to when or if I would need to tell anyone outside of the room we were currently in.

The second person I mentioned this information to was Kris Maassen. She is an amazing woman whom I also met and connected with at work. Let me state that for me, she became my mentor the first time I laid eyes on her in my beginnings with this new company. I hadn't asked her, just made a decision that through her words, her presence, her knowledge that she was a God-given person that could drive, motivate, and push me. Being a two-time survivor, I knew Kris would pour into me, so if I wanted advice from anyone on what to expect during the process and questions I should be asking, I knew her voice mattered to me.

I reached out to her on the day of the biopsy when I was working from home and asked her if I could have a few minutes. She said, "Absolutely," and my feelings at that moment only screamed out, "Blessed!"

When I got Kris on the phone, the conversation started casually, and then I took the dive. "So I asked for this meeting because I have something personal going on and really would like your thoughts on how I should approach it. I found a lump."

She stopped me and said, "Hold on, let me close my office door." And at that moment, our relationship shifted from mentor/mentee to survivor coach and student. She was transparent, kind, compassionate, and amazingly supportive. We talked through where I was in the process. I explained that the biopsy was scheduled and I was scared. She told me what to expect. "It will be painful, but you've got this, and I'm here for you, whatever you need," she said. She encouraged me to keep her posted, let her know what was going on, and let me know that she was praying for me. I cried, and she cried with me. She shared her story in detail not once but twice. She'd endured this fight, and she was now a ten-year survivor living, loving, giving, and beautiful!

My biopsy took place at the SSM Cancer Center in St. Peters, Missouri, about twenty minutes from home. When it was time for biopsy, I walked into the building with my hubby hand in hand. He was smiling and being his annoying self in an attempt to keep me calm, levelheaded, and providing just the support I needed! We walked in, and the receptionist greeted us with love and concern. She was an extremely gentle spirit, super kind and amazing. What was different about this experience was it felt like she felt my fear. She prayed with me and told me I would be fine.

Since I was back a second time, she remembered me. I'm almost certain she knew why I was there. She came back over to me after I checked in while we were sitting and handed me a card, gave me a big hug, and told me that I had this and God was already in control! Her card was beautiful. It touched my soul, and again I cried. This day was super-emotional, if you hadn't gotten that already.

They called my name, and I gave hubby a kiss and walked back to change into that awful open front wraparound shirt that provides no warmth in the cold hospital setting. The nurse came back to get me once I had changed and walked me into the room where the procedure would be completed. The doctor and the lab tech begin on my right side, first scanning the area to detect where they would take the sample of the mass. Nurse Becky came over to the bed and grabbed my hand. As tears began falling down the sides of my face, she kept holding my hand as it was lifted over my head. She rubbed my arm and kept encouraging me to take deep breaths while giving me positive affirmations that it would be okay and to hang in there.

Although I didn't know her, I needed her and needed those words at that moment. "Okay, Anastasia, I'm going to stick the needle in, and you'll hear a pretty loud snap that will let you know that I have taken the sample."

That crap hurts! Nothing like a needle going into your breast collecting samples and letting you know it's doing so by a loud *snap* at the time of collection. They then moved over to my left side. This time, the doctor said since there were three masses. She would try to obtain them in two sticks instead of sticking me three times. She was successful in the two sticks, although the sticking and collecting hurt! The process took about an hour and a half to obtain all four samples! At the conclusion, I asked, "So what's the best guess from what you've seen? They're all benign, right?"

And with a solid demeanor that I wasn't ready for, Nurse Becky declared she was about 90 percent positive that the three on the left were cancerous.

I again tried my optimism. "But they could be benign."

And she repeated with the same solid, stern demeanor, "I cannot agree with you, they look cancerous."

Usually, men were not allowed to come back in this area of the building, but because it was later in the evening, there were no other women waiting for a procedure, scan, mammogram, or ultrasound, Nurse Becky went to get Corey. When he walked in, he sat down on a stool in front of me, and all I recall at that moment was my head hitting his chest with a force that I was sure had knocked the wind out of him. Tears were streaming down my face, but in the back of my mind, I thought, *She doesn't have the final say!*

From there, Nurse Becky invited us into her office where my mom joined us. With tissues in hand, she told me that she knew how I felt as she too had been through this process and have overcome the beast that is breast cancer. We began talking about next steps, but in the meantime, as we were talking, she started putting together a pink and white "SSM Healthcare Breast Cancer" bag. In it, there was a pink and white breast cancer blanket. She added some books for myself, the kids, Corey, and my other caretakers to read and discuss. The bag also held a beanie for when I lost my hair and a small pillow to place under my arm to relieve some of the pain from the biopsy sites on my left side.

I don't remember the questions I asked or that Corey asked. I remember thinking, "Is she so positive that I have cancer that she is giving me this bag of stuff? I think we're jumping the gun a bit!" I never said it out loud, but it felt like a closed case situation.

As we finished, she gave me a hug and told me I was going to be fine, that the road ahead would suck but I will overcome this issue. We left the building, and all I could do was cry, but I needed to get myself under control because shortly, we'd be picking up the kids.

On Friday, February 22, I got the call. The doctor said what we all pray never to hear. "Hi, Anastasia. This is Dr. Vaughan calling from the SSM Cancer treatment center. I'm sorry to let you know I've gotten your preliminary results, and I can confirm that the three tumors in your left breast are cancer, the one on the right is benign. I'm so sorry. I know this isn't what you wanted to hear, but I wanted to get the results to you before the weekend as I had promised."

Dr. Vaughan had dropped the bomb! And while I heard the rest of the conversation, I wasn't listening. Something about the nurse would be calling to schedule the next appointments and we'd go through the information and blah, blah, blah! *What in the world? I have cancer! Why? Why me, God? What did I do to deserve this? What about my husband and kids? Is this it? Will this kill me? I have cancer. I really have cancer!* Major blow.

I turned to look at Corey, and it was safe to say he knew. What I love about my husband is his eyes. No matter what the situation is, his eyes tell the truth. When I finally made eye contact, he stared back at me. He told me it would be okay, better than okay. He told me I was strong and that we would get through this thing together. He told me this didn't change his love for me and that we'd grow through this thing. And his eyes told me that was all true, but it did not stop the emotional floodgates that had been cranked open.

The next step was to begin telling people. I knew I would need support, encouragement, and big-time love through this. I knew there were some important people that needed to know to stand with me, to pray for me, and to pray for my family. The first stop was my mom. Mom had kept the kids for us, so they knew nothing, and I wanted to shelter them a little while longer. When Corey and I got to my mom's house, I tried to keep it light. A normal conversation about the kids and the family and the pleasantries. She had cooked, which was a good and a bad thing. I mean, who doesn't love their mom's food? But how could I eat when I had this bomb I was about to drop? I figured I'd get a little and sit down to chat, and that's what I did.

At the end of the plate, Corey and I made eye contact. "Mom, I need to tell you something," I proceeded. I gave her the rundown, and then I said, "I have breast cancer."

Her demeanor immediately weakened. I believe this is the type of hurt that no parent wants to feel, the feelings of "There is nothing I can do to stop this, change it, or make it go away." I felt her pain. It was long and deep. I continued, "But we are going to fight, keep the faith, and this too shall pass!" I said it with confidence, yet tears started to fall.

She began to cry and she held me. She said she was so sorry, and like all mothers…she knew something wasn't right. She felt it before the words leaped from my lips. Mother's intuition, I guess. We discussed it—what it meant, the doctors I had chosen (or had chosen me), and my plan of attack. She reassured that she would be in this fight with me and would be wherever or whatever I needed her to be. After a while, Corey and I packed up the kids and we went home. I felt like a heavy load had been lifted. We had been carrying this for two weeks on our own, and now the secret was out. Now what?

CaringBridge Entry: It's Becoming Real
Journal entry by Anastasia Stevenson—
March 12, 2019

Today is almost surreal. I'm doing things around the house to prep for and attempting to embrace my new normal! I've scheduled work around the house, I've scheduled a hair appointment and scheduled a family portrait session. My mom will take the kids this weekend so that Corey and I can spend some time together. I have an education appointment this Friday to understand my chemo meds and how to take care of my port. I'm looking around and thinking, *Wow, this is actually happening in real life.* I'm nervous but not scared; I'm ready but feel unprepared…it is feels crazy!

My port is scheduled to be put in on Monday, March 18th, and my first session of chemo is March 19th! The past month has been a whirlwind, and yet here we are… I'm still standing, and I will continue to do so.

Special shout-outs to my hubby, my mom, my brother, Jerry, & SIL Lucy & two closest friends, Zundra and Brandi! I would not have gotten this far without you. Thank you for loving me through my tears and fears and for standing when I was too weak. I love you all to the moon and back!

Out for now!
Anastasia

Chapter 2

The Diagnosis and the Plan

"For I know the plans I have for you," declares
the Lord. "Plans to prosper you and not to harm
you, plans to give you hope and a future."
—Jeremiah 29:11 (NIV)

It has been said that trials come to make us stronger, and for the most part, they do; but what happens when that trial is a decision to live or die? It seemed that this was the crossroad that I was facing. The doctor asked me very plainly, "Anastasia, do you want to fight or do you want to die?"

In truth, this story really began two months before I found the lump in my left breast. On a Wednesday night Bible study, Pastor David Blunt of Church on the Rock in St. Peters, Missouri, was ending his sermon. He asked, "What will we believe God for in 2019? What would we trust Him to do in our lives?"

That sat with me for a while, and I felt as if Pastor was speaking directly to me—it was one of those types of sermons. I took action simply because "Faith without work is dead" (James 2:26). I sowed a seed of faith and committed to completing the twenty-one-day fast with the church beginning the first week of January 2019. I came home excited and had complete joy and expectancy from the decision that I had made at church. I told Corey about it and got him onboard to join me in the fast. I decided my answer to Pastor's question regarding what I would trust God to do in 2019 were as follows:

1. Rebuild my marriage on a solid foundation. Corey and I were struggling in our marriage for a number of reasons. There was a wall of trust that needed to be rebuilt and restored. We needed to understand what it meant to be in love with each other and put each other first, no matter what and fallback in love—you know, the puppy dog love we have in the earlier parts of our relationships. We needed to tear down and rebuild.

2. Be the example and help lead my children to Christ. After all, he only allowed us to borrow them until such time as they are called back home to be with him. More than that, I wanted our family to be different, break generational curses, and show our children what faith in God, Jesus, and the Holy Spirit looked like. "I needed a *lot* more Jesus"—in my best Erica Campbell voice!

3. My next thing was to reunite my broken family. Many of us come from families that have, in some way, been

broken down and torn apart. My aunts and uncles aren't in a healthy relationship with each other nor my mom. I am the youngest of ten children—seven brothers and two sisters—and before you ask, no, my mom did not give birth to all of those kids. My dad had seven children with his wife who had passed away before he met my mom. While we all love each other, some of us have better relationships than others, and I was sick of that!

4. Finally, and probably most importantly, I wanted to have God heal the hurts of my past. As a child, I'd been molested more than once. I'd wrecked the relationship between myself and my mom because I was so much of a "Daddy's girl." I blamed her for his passing. I'd fallen in love and had my heart broken in my late teens and dropped out of college. I'd been abused in a relationship and had to go back to live with my mom. Things happened, and while I survived, I stuffed them and made myself move on without acknowledging or getting help. I've been diagnosed with depression and anxiety, and I brought all of this into my relationship, now married to my husband. It was time to let go, heal, and move forward.

As the New Year rolled around, I leaned fully into the fast, giving up caffeine (which was a *big* deal as I had a small addiction to Pepsi and my daily Starbucks go-to was a white chocolate mocha with whole milk, whipped cream, and two shots of caramel)! I also decided to give up sweets—this was a hefty goal! However, for the list of things I wanted God to move in, I needed to make some major sacrifices! I started out well. I had great intentions and tons of hope and awesome support! About a week in, my husband started slacking, but I kept going strong. I was committed, but I completely overlooked that this was my first missed opportunity to bring Corey and I closer together.

Around day sixteen, I nudged him and asked him to finish strong with me...day sixteen! He agreed, and we began sharing our daily journals with each other before bed. Mine were extended stories while his were a sentence or two—straightforward and to the point. I guess it's true that women use more words than men daily, but I wouldn't, shouldn't, and couldn't complain because he was participating and was not complaining about doing so.

We finished the twenty-one days and were off to learning to communicate, being better to and for each other, even agreeing to pay more attention to each other while keeping God at the center of our relationship. But then life happened! In the last quarter of the year, I enrolled in a doctoral program. I figured I had the ability to stay on top of things at home with Corey and the kids (inclusive of after-school sports and activities), be a great daughter, sister, and friend, continue to climb the corporate ladder, be on nonprofit boards, *and* obtain a Ph.D. My focus on the things I said I wanted in the beginning of the year shifted, and I can't even tell you when I began putting those four priorities on the back burner. I prayed, asked for forgiveness, and to be put back on the right track...and then the lump was found. I felt as if this began a new test of what I would trust—the word and works of the doctors alone, the words and thoughts that were in my mind, or *the* Word and my heavenly Father.

After confirmation of my diagnosis, things began moving pretty quickly. I had a few phone calls from nurses that would be planning the next steps to get me ready for treatment.

I would have a port-a-cath placed, a chemo education meeting with a nurse practitioner, a meeting at the chemo center to see where chemo would happen, meet a few of the nurses, see a nutritionist, and ultimately meet my oncologist. I also needed to begin telling my diagnosis to my immediate friends and family. I would also inform my team at work.

I'd decided who would and would not be told by me because the news would eventually get out. I also decided to take a hiatus from social media. I did not want a bunch of "so-called sympathy" from folks who really didn't and don't care about my family or circumstances. In my short life, I've learned that some folks tend to want bad things to happen to you so that they can feel better about themselves. I removed that extra layer of nothing from my life.

I had decided early on that the year 2019 would be about intentionality, doing nothing wastefully, and embracing myself wholly. All of this had gotten me to a place of being completely overwhelmed. I had done one of the things that Nurse Becky pressed me not to do, which was Google, YouTube, and conduct endless searches on breast cancer. I did exactly that, and everything that I came across was negative, especially about chemo. I had a full-on breakdown.

My husband was not able to console me and called one of my best friends. Her name is Zundra. I don't know what he said to her, but he handed me the phone. She asked if I needed her to come over, and my answer was yes. When she got to the house, I was in a complete bawling session in my bathroom. She came in, opened the door, pulled me up, and brought me to the couch. She held me close and asked me to listen to her breath to help me calm down. I did as I was instructed until my babbling "ugly cry" was toned down to a whimper, but tears were still falling.

She asked me questions like what I was thinking, and my response was, "What if I die! What if I leave my family, my babies? What if I'm not strong enough to get through this?"

She calmly said, "Anastasia, you still have work to do. What about those young ladies you want to impact? What about God taking care of you and your family? What about all of the love you still have to give? What about all of those things?"

My cry settled a little more. Corey came back to the room, seemingly happy but also frustrated. "She would never have calmed down that easily for me." He was, although shamefully, absolutely right. This was another opportunity in our marriage to be vulnerable with each other and let the other person's words take root.

Zundra, having been married for over twenty years, shed some light on that thing. We had additional dialog about allowing myself to be truly naked with Corey because he would be the backbone of the operation from here on out. Yes, I would have other support, but Corey was it! I needed him, and he needed me to allow him in to be part of the process and embrace this whole situation together. That was so much easier said than done, but I agreed and promised him I would work on it.

The following day, I heard from Zundra again, just checking in on me to see if it was a better day. I told her yes but that I still struggled with it a little. She confirmed that it was totally normal and to give myself some grace to feel everything that I felt. This would become a common mantra for me throughout this process. What came next was her asking what I needed. I didn't know, but she began probing. "Do you want to get some people together to just be together?"

And I replied, "A headwrap party." Now I don't know where this thought came from, but I figured if I'd be losing my hair, having a few head wraps would be a good thing. She agreed and asked if she should engage anyone else. "Yes," I replied, "Brandi, my bestie of over twenty years."

She simply said okay and to give her a date and a list of names with phone numbers or e-mail addresses, and they'd handle the rest.

The following week, I worked from home to get a handle on things and attend a few appointments. I scheduled a home-cleaning to sanitize the house, a duct-cleaning to remove dirt, allergens, and such from our cooling/heating system, took the kids to their dental appointments, scheduled my own dental appointment (per the request of the doctor because I would not be able to have these during chemo treatment), made a hair appointment, and scheduled a family portrait session to capture "normal" life with my family before any of this changed.

Digging a little deeper into the acts that I had begun doing to take care of home, I realized that I was also doing another type of preparation. The pictures, the hair, and the normal I spoke about were all out of fear—the fear that I would not be around very much longer. I had, in my own mind, sentenced myself to live a very short life. The pictures would be a reminder for my children of the strength their mother had in her wholeness before cancer decided to show up. My husband wouldn't need to look for a photo of me for the obituary, and my family could see a big gorgeous smile instead of whatever cancer would do to my skin and weight. I was selfishly and secretly planning my demise.

This week would also include Brandi's birthday celebration. So another good girlfriend and I planned a dinner with a few small surprises. It gave me a chance to relax and not think about what would be happening in the next few weeks and also gave me (a project manager by profession) a chance to prepare, plan, and put things in order. Brandi and I met up early in the morning as she would be accompanying me to my chemo education meeting, and being the wonderful friend that she is, she also picked up breakfast. We went to the chemo center and went into the education room where the nurse practitioner (NP) would be giving a rundown on my meds, my schedule, potential side effects, recipe books, and a whole lot more.

Brandi took notes while the NP talked. We talked about the medicines, treatment cycles, and side effects. We walked over into the chemotherapy room where we would meet one of the nurses that would help in providing me treatment. Her name was Jeannie. She was a light-spirited woman with dark hair and stood about five-foot-five (I only mention her height because I'm about five-foot-nine and feel as though I tower over her). I shook her hand, and she said very proudly and reassuringly that she was going to take very good care of me, and instantly, without a pause, a flood of emotions washed over me. I was in tears in the arms of a woman I didn't know in the last place I thought I would ever be. *How could this be happening? What does this mean? Why me?* She continued to rub my back and handed me a Kleenex. She assured me that this would be temporary and would fly by, "but I promise to take good care of you."

I get a little more information, and we began walking to the exit. As I mentioned previously, this was my best friend's birthday weekend, so I had booked a float spa after this appointment to relax for an hour. I think we both needed it at this moment. We grabbed our stuff and headed out to the car. I was quiet, and she was looking over at me. "Sta (as she calls me), what are you thinking? Are you okay?"

I did my usual, "Yes, I'm good. Let's head over to the spa. Follow me." We get in our cars, and I called Corey. "Babe, I'm scared."

Typical him said, "We'll be okay, I got you, bae. Just head over to the spa and relax. We'll talk it all out this evening. I want to know everything." His voice was calming and reassuring. I'm not sure Corey knew how pivotal he was in pulling me through all of this.

Brandi and I pulled into the lot at the float spa and prepared to be lost in a quiet world for a little while, just take a break from it all and lean into the peacefulness of the experience before us. I'm grateful she was with me and held me up with light laughter, a smile, and the peace of her presence. We go into our separate spa rooms and into the warm salted water. I retreat in prayer. "Jesus, I don't know how I will get through this. I need you now. Take over, lead, and guide me. Let me feel your love and your healing presence. I declare that I am healed in Jesus's name. By your stripes, I am healed (Isaiah 53:5). Amen." And then I closed my eyes and drifted off, shut down my thoughts, and allowed the water and salt to carry me to dreamland.

> CaringBridge Entry: One Week…Lots of Change
> Journal entry by Anastasia Stevenson—March 23, 2019
>
> This week was a tough one. This is where the rubber met the road. On Monday, I had the outpatient procedure to have my port put in. On Tuesday, I had my first chemotherapy treatment. My emotions were of course all over the place. I've cried out, prayed, been angry and so much more!
>
> Immediately following chemo, I felt pretty good. But that soon took a turn. On

Wednesday evening I was transported via ambulance to the Emergency room to help alleviate some pain, control the nausea and get hydrated. This week this has turned life upside down several times!

How are the kids?! They are resilient, persistent and as long as there are food and snacks and the play park, everyone is adjusting. CJ is asking questions yet being extremely thoughtful, concerned and helpful.

Corey Sr. is amazing! My backbone and source of energy. He's a blessing every single day. I've had tons of people calling, texting, stopping by and video chatting to check on me...from the bottom of my heart...*thank you!*

I Love you *all!*

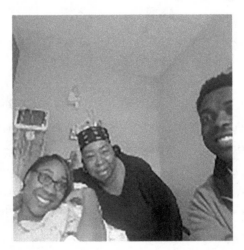

From left to right, Anastasia, Anastasia's mom Eloise and Husband Corey pre-surgery to place port and the day before chemo began

Anastasia and Corey outside of the Cancer Treatment center on the first day of chemo

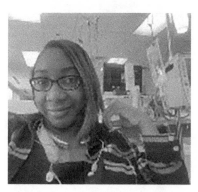

Anastasia seated and preparing to get started with chemo

Chapter 3

Acceptance & Denial

Be strong and of good courage, fear not, nor be afraid of them: for the Lord thy God, it is He that goes with thee; he will not fail thee nor forsake thee.
—Deuteronomy 31:6 (ESV)

You know, it's extremely difficult to walk through the wilderness of a new diagnosis in that it will completely alter life as I know it. Let me acknowledge that while things were not perfect, I had been living a beautiful life. I was the first of my immediate sisters and brothers to obtain a higher education degree, let alone two master's degrees, I had an amazing husband and three wonderful healthy children. We lived in a really nice home that Corey and I built from the ground up as first-time homeowners shortly after we were married in 2009. I also had a great job that allowed me to remain active in the community and continue my learning and development. I had great friends and some supportive family. That was more than enough. I was extremely blessed. But who could expect, want, or even think that something like this would impact them? Breast cancer. And then I thought, *Well, why not? I'm no different than any other wife, mom, daughter, sister, or friend that has been diagnosed with this disease.*

I pondered on why this might have happened to me. I was not an easy teenager to deal with, especially after the death of my father. I was not the best wife. I'd hurt my husband and didn't want to really acknowledge that. I didn't think I was the best mom because I spent time outside of our house, networking and trying to build my career. I had been selfish, and maybe this was my payback for that. Maybe I owed it to the universe to get it right since I had been so "negative" in the past. I took the burden and made it all about the wrong thing, shifting the focus away from my family and feeling sorry for myself. Lying in a pit of ugliness that separated me from my family even more, I cried, screamed, was angry, and simply mean. I shut down and began sinking more and more inward to myself.

All of us digest bad news, even good news for that matter, differently. We don't take the time to think objectively or derive some type of good outlook from the situation. As I am a woman of faith, I think my response was supposed to be an immediate cry out to Jesus to turn it all over because I had complete confidence in him, but it wasn't. And guess what? That's okay. I'm not perfect, and I don't know why we put so much emphasis on trying to be when we can only handle what is in front of us. We try to manipulate and control things and situations, but it wasn't until breast cancer that I realized I was never in control. That's a hard realization and a tough thing to accept.

Like anyone receiving bad news, I had to digest the information and then determine what to do with it. I knew I needed to take action, but what type of action? I went through a period of denial. Not me, not now. Now is where I was working on my doctoral degree and I had put myself on a timeline to complete it. I did not have time to deal with this type of negativity in my life! Now was the time that I needed to continue the education process with my children. This was a pivotal age, and I needed to be here and present for this. I did not have time for cancer. Now was the time for me to do lots of networking to build my career so that I could continue to elevate and climb the corporate ladder. I could not do that with cancer on my plate! I simply could not and would not accept this horrible fate.

Needless to say, that was a short-lived soapbox moment because the tears of reality began to flow as I received continual calls to book appointments with doctors that I knew nothing about. The wheels began turning so quickly that I had to make a decision to fight. After all, this was a real thing that I needed to deal with before it dealt with me. My cancer was described as Stage 2B IDC. That's a fancy way of saying that the cancer tumors that were present in my left breast, three in total, were between two to five millimeters in size and had begun to spread from the milk ducts in my breast to the lymph nodes underneath my arm.

In addition to this news, Dr. Vaughan made me aware that one of the tumors was directly behind my areola, and when it was time, I would need to think about and perhaps face the fact that I would need to have my entire nipple and areola removed. If that mass did not decrease in size from the chemo, and even if it did, she didn't want the risk of it recurring in that spot. Additionally, if we took one, we might as well take both.

In appointment after appointment, I had to listen, take in the information, and decide what to do with it. For many of those appointments, I had reinforcements that proved to be necessary and critical in helping me digest the information I had been given and even recall some of it. They took notes, asked questions that I couldn't think of, recorded the sessions so that I could go back and listen to them and, most importantly, held my hand and handed me tissues. It seemed almost every appointment had some shedding of tears. I had a flood of thoughts from wondering how I would tackle this and still manage the things on my plate to will this be the end of me? Will this disease take me from my husband and children, what will their lives be like without me? These are real questions that cross our minds, real questions that sometimes we believe we have the answers to, and other times, we are almost certainly uncertain.

Denial came upon me as I would go home and look at myself in the mirror and think, *I don't look sick!* I felt normal with the normal aches and pains and headaches of life. I realized I had low energy from being an active mom and wife, but that was normal. You know, the days of dropping off at school, driving to work, picking up from school, going to some after school activity, heading to church, then going home for baths and bed, cleaning the kitchen in the evening or throwing in a load of laundry—the normal life. The only abnormal thing was this knot in my breast— well, three knots that I knew weren't supposed to be there.

I circled back and forth in my mind, wondering what I did to bring this upon myself. Was it because I had so many blocked duct issues while breastfeeding the twins? Was it my diet or fluctuating weight? Was it the start and stop of the times I exercised? Was it truly genetics that had taken a wrong turn within me? Or had I just done so much damage in my past that this was God's way of paying me back for all the horrible things I had done in my life? These were real questions I posed to myself, wondering how I could have been such a bad person that God would choose me to give this disease to. *This is the way I needed to learn a lesson? Really, God?*

Here again is where I struggled because I knew that the God I claimed to serve would not give me a disease. If I knew nothing else, it was that it was time for me to activate the faith within, to begin to stand on the promise of his Word. I needed to make a decision, a choice as to what I believed would be my fate, and make that decision quickly.

> *I have said these things to you, that you may have peace. In the world, you will have tribulation. But take heart, I have over-come the world. (John 16:33 ESV)*

Details regarding the headwrap party were still being determined. I hadn't provided a vision. I trusted Brandi and Zundra for that. Zundra had begun sending me the regrets of those that would not be able to make it to the party but still left messages of love, faith, hope, and healing—words that I would later rely on to keep me going through the journey.

A few days later, on March 18, I was scheduled to have surgery to have my port (a small, implantable reservoir with a thin silicone tube that attaches to a vein) placed. The main advantage of this vein-access device is that chemotherapy medications can be delivered directly into the port rather than a vein, eliminating the need for needle sticks and the potential of blowing veins due to the amount and toxicity of the medications that would soon be entering my body. This was an outpatient procedure that would be conducted by my breast surgeon, Dr. Alison Vaughan of the SSM Cancer Medical Care Team in St. Peters, Missouri. Dr. Vaughan is at the top of her field in the St. Louis region and is an amazing doctor. I am extremely blessed to be within her care.

The surgery went smoothly, and I was in and out in about an hour. Dr. Vaughan said that she would leave my port accessed (keep the needle in) in preparation for my first chemotherapy (chemo) session that was scheduled for the following day, March 19, bright and early at 9:00 a.m. I left the hospital loopy but okay.

I began to feel sore later on that night but remedied the pain with the prescribed pain medications. I tried to sleep, but there was none of that happening. I was anxious about what chemo would feel like and how I would feel, because according to the pamphlets I kept reading over and over, there was a huge possibility that I would be absolutely miserable!

The headwrap party was held a few days after the port had been put in and also a few days after my first chemo treatment, which we'll talk about in the next chapter. The party was a complete experience. I had no idea what Zundra and Brandi had told the list of attendees that were coming to the party. I didn't even know who had accepted and who had not. I was only told to arrive fashionably late, which is touch for me because I'm usually on time, if not early, for any and every event that I attend.

Upon my arrival, I saw many cars, way more than I expected to see there. For some reason, I had made up the story in my mind that there wouldn't be many people there because they had better things to do than to attend yet another "typical" Saturday party. This thing was anything but typical. I had the conversation with Brandi and Zundra that I would be wearing a mask due to my compromised immune system. The chemo drugs tended to have that effect. Again, we'll talk about that in the next chapter.

I felt weird and thought that the people that had shown up would think it was weird too, but that was the trick of the enemy. When I walked in, I was received with love, hugs, and smiles. The house was full, and people were everywhere, scattered from the kitchen to the living room, over into the dining room. I had sisters, aunts, and cousins, co-workers—including my boss, Laura—prayer partners, close friends, and of course, my mom—such a remarkable feeling. Zundra and Brandi agreed that this would be a woman's only event, so my husband, brothers, and any other men in my life were not allowed to be present. This is something that you need to be able to feel what you feel, and no one is uncomfortable about the discussion and topic at hand.

What I was not aware of was that I was told to be late so that Brandi and Zundra could update everyone in the room on where I was in the process, what the diagnosis was, and answer any of the questions they could to relieve me from that duty once I arrived. When I got there, I was not consumed with the what, how, when, what's next questions. That had been taken care of for me, and I'm so grateful that they took that weight off of me. It's a heavy burden to carry and a lot of information to provide over and over again.

We ate, we laughed, and we loved each other. About an hour into the gathering, Zundra suggested that we open the wraps, and again, I didn't have great expectations, but oh my goodness! Everyone brought a wrap, and some brought more than one. Each one was different. As a matter of fact, of all of the wraps I opened, only one was a duplicate. I read the cards, and most brought me to tears. I tried to hold my composure and continue going through these beautiful wraps of many colors, sizes, and textures. I counted seventy-three wraps in total!

What came next absolutely took me by surprise. Brandi had pulled one of the photos she had of me and had them printed in four-by-six photo sheets, and on the bottom of each picture, there were words like *Survivor, Warrior,* etc.; and on the back of each picture, the women in attendance had written me a note. These were gathered together and put in a small box. The box was given to me, and I was told that I was to use these when I needed just a little more strength to get through some of the rough days that may be ahead.

After that, we went into prayer. People from around the room would just jump in to say their prayer for me. That moment led to an all-out outcry to heaven, singing "Break Every Chain" by Grammy-winning artist Tasha Cobbs. The room was so full, some crying, others in full out praise! It was absolutely amazing! To be loved in that way is something I will never forget and highly encourage! Sometimes you just have to let go and surrender to the will of Jesus.

Turns out, this part of the party wasn't planned, but it worked out for all of our good. All I could get out at the end of all of that was I was going to fight, no matter what I would go through or how hard it got. For those prayers, that support, those tears, and that outcry, I knew I needed to forge forward in the road that was before me.

That day, I felt overwhelmed with love, positivity, and grace. As we packed up the scarves and the people and began to leave the house, all with tight embraces encouraging words, I could feel my heartbeat. It felt as if I had run upstairs and ran back down. I now know that my internal was matching the thoughts running through my mind a million thoughts per second. I was appreciative, joyful, and also heartbroken. My heart broke for the people that were hurting for me, that were nervous for me, but were also in the fight with me.

It was at this point that denial was completely out of the door. I was now what I would call in full swing of moving forward on an operation that I called "Operation Get It the Hell *Out!*" This to me was the significant moment of acceptance that this was happening to me whether I wanted it to or not and whether I agreed or not.

CaringBridge Entry: Thank You
Journal entry by Anastasia Stevenson—
March 25, 2019

I could not go another 24 hours without saying thank you! The women God has surrounded me with are so amazing. To have my family with me on this journey is exactly what I need! You are my family.

The only word that I still have is Grateful! I'm so grateful for the love, support, prayers, prayer warriors, peace, understanding, transparency and joy that you all bring. You made Saturday exactly what I needed it to be! You covered me!

This evening I sat and started reading some of the beautiful love notes you wrote and I'm speechless. Tears have flowed…tears of rejoice and reverence to God for the village that is you…all of you!

Zundra and Brandi, words cannot express how thankful I am for you. You are amazing and I'm so blessed to know you, love you and call you my sisters! I sincerely thank you for

all the work you put into Saturday and every-
day you've spent with me from the beginning
of this up through and beyond the all clear!

Thank you, thank you, thank you! I love
you!

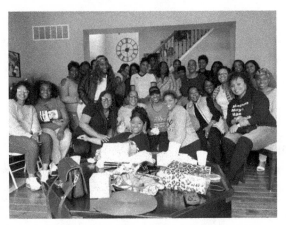

Anastasia's village at the head wrap party...
this isn't the entire village!

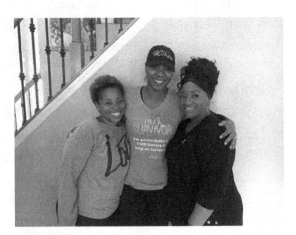

From left to right, Zundra, Anastasia & Brandi at the head
wrap party. They are more than friends, my sisters.

CaringBridge Entry: Figuring it Out
Journal entry by Anastasia Stevenson—Mar 27, 2019

Hey Family,

Today we had an opportunity to figure out some things. I'm learning about my medicine! Today's event included a trip to the ER. We learned that some of the meds that I'm on have side effects that include horrible muscle spasms and bone pain. The SSM team did well in making assessments, running tests and checking to be sure there were no stones left unturned. I'm still having some pain but doing much better than this morning.

On another note, on Sunday my scalp had begun to burn and become extremely uncomfortable. This was a sign that my hair would begin shedding. On Monday, running my fingers through my hair would bring me to tears…my hair was coming out! I thought I had another few weeks…not so much! After talking with Corey, we decided that this is something that we would control! I called my good girlfriend over to hold my hand on Tuesday night to make the change! As I cried, Kanisha held my hand and Corey took the clippers and cut my hair!

So how do I feel??? I feel free, a little unsure but mostly empowered! The best thing that happened that night was as soon as Kennedi and Aaliyah saw it they said "Mommy's pretty, I want to cut my hair, too!" How that blessed my soul, I was speechless!

Thank you Kanisha for holding my hand, for your encouragement, for standing with me and calling me beautiful! You, my friend, are amazing and beautiful inside and out!

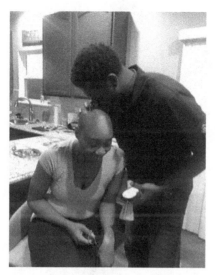

Corey kissing Anastasia's head after shaving hair

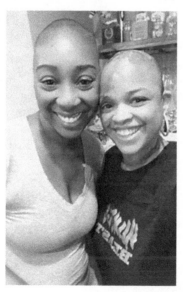

Anastasia & Kanisha Anthony. Kanisha wiped tears, documented
the moment and was a complete support in cutting off my hair.

Chapter 4

Medication, Radiation, and Surgeries—Oh My!

But He was wounded for our transgressions, He was bruised for our iniquities, the chastisement for our peace was upon Him. And by His stripes, we are healed.
—Isaiah 53:5 (ESV)

When all would be said and done, according to the doctors, I would have sixteen rounds of chemo with four different drugs, twenty-eight rounds of radiation, and four surgeries. What I knew was that this situation was different for every survivor that had been diagnosed with this disease. In my experience, I completed chemo before taking on surgery or radiation. The order, amount, and frequency are person and doctor-specific and are based on your case and your case alone. There is not a one-size fits all approach! In this portion of the book, I'll be describing the medications and approach used in my case. I am *not* a licensed health practitioner, and you should *not* by any stretch of the imagination base your care or your loved ones' care on my experience.

Now that is out of the way, let's dig into the details. I solidified who my doctors would be within the SSM Cancer Health Group. Dr. Vaughan would be my breast surgeon, Dr. Pascale Salem would be my medical oncologist, Dr. Anna Fu my radiation oncologist, and Dr. Paul Mills (Renaissance Plastic Surgery) my plastic surgeon. Dr. Vaughan let me know that this team would be chatting on my progress and discussing the best continuation of treatment throughout my journey. I knew it held true because every meeting I had with any of those doctors, they knew what the plan was without me speaking.

The necessary alignment and order of process and procedure was clearly discussed, and everyone was on the same page. For me, this provided a sense of relief and a knowing that God was in control. I had not heard of such synchronization in other women's experiences. The doctors were well-acquainted with each other's styles and aligned their techniques for their patients.

I met with each doctor prior to beginning treatment to outline the plan, come into consensus, and understand the path. Not all information was divulged in those meetings for my own benefit. I would receive the information that would be pertinent for me to know, and as I approached each residual phase, more information would be provided. Though my journey began with Dr. Vaughan, the work would begin with Dr. Salem, the chemo doctor.

Dr. Salem was a rather small woman. I towered over her in height. She had a small voice, but her outer demeanor gave me confidence and was extremely encouraging. Her staff and other medical techs that I'd had the pleasure of meeting upon visits confirmed that I was in great hands. They said that she was absolutely one of the best in her field and took her work personally. I could glean this to be true as we started our rather frequent visits.

~Chemotherapy~

On March 19, as scheduled, Corey and I pulled into the parking lot of the St. Joseph Cancer Center parking lot. He was armed with my bag that contained a blanket, a journal, ink pen, extra change of underwear (you can never be too prepared), headphones, nausea medicine, and my cell phone. In addition, he had his work backpack, which held his laptop, a notebook, and a couple of pens.

Before we walked in, we snapped a selfie, and I took a shot of the front of the building. My stomach was in knots, and I had zero expectations. We were by far the youngest people in the waiting room. I signed in and waited for them to call my name. Shortly thereafter, I heard, "Anastasia."

They told Corey to sit tight. They started by just taking my labs, and I'd be back out and then called to see Dr. Salem, and she'd escort me to the infusion room. The lab technician was quick and efficient. Seemingly stuck, drawn, and wrapped up in a single swoop, I went back out to join Corey, and again I heard, "Anastasia."

This time I would see Dr. Salem. We began the conversation with the normal things. She reviewed my lab work and then took a look at me. We began walking through the medicines again, this time at a very high level, ensuring she highlighted the side effects.

Dr. Salem was clear that we would be very aggressive with the cycle of medicines that she prescribed. She felt as if we needed to grab the bull by the horns and to do everything we could to decrease the chance of the cancer ever returning. She explained that the first grouping of medicines I would be on would be Adriamycin (lovingly nicknamed the red devil), Cytoxan, and Neulasta. These would be given over four treatments every other week. Then we'd move on to Taxol that would be given weekly for twelve weeks. We again discussed the side effects of each. They went something like this:

"The first three medicines, you may experience some or all of these to some extent. Adriamycin is used to treat different types of cancers that affect the breast, bladder, kidneys, ovaries, thyroid, stomach, lungs, bones, nerve tissues, joints, and soft tissues. Adriamycin can weaken your immune system. Your blood is tested weekly, and you should tell me if you have unusual bruising or bleeding or signs of infection (fever, chills, body aches). Adriamycin may cause dangerous effects on your heart. Call me if you feel very weak or tired or have fast heartbeats, shortness of breath (even with mild exertion), or swelling in your ankles or feet. It may also cause early menopause (good thing we had made the decision that our family was complete).

"Avoid being near people who are sick or have infections. Call me if you develop signs of infection and fevers. Avoid activities that may increase your risk of bleeding or injury. Use extra care to prevent bleeding while shaving or brushing your teeth.

This medicine can pass into body fluids (urine, feces, vomit). For at least forty hours, after you receive a dose, avoid allowing your body fluids to come into contact with your hands or other surfaces. Your caregivers should wear rubber gloves when cleaning up any body fluids.

"Make sure to wash hands before and after removing gloves. Wash all of your clothing and linens separately from other laundry. During treatment, if you feel dizzy, nauseated, light-headed, sweaty, or have a headache, chest tightness, back pain, trouble breathing, or swelling in your face, tell the nurses right away as you may be having an allergic reaction to the medicine, but we will give you premeds before we start your regimen to attempt to prevent this. The list of side effects from this medicine include pain, blisters, or skin sores where the injection was given, missed menstrual periods, easy bruising, unusual bleeding, low white blood cell counts—fever, swollen gums, painful mouth sores, pain when swallowing, skin sores, cold or flu symptoms, cough, trouble breathing, signs of heart problems—fast heartbeats, shortness of breath (even with mild exertion), feeling very weak or tired, swelling in your ankles or feet, your urine to turn a reddish-orange color. Also, nausea, vomiting, and hair loss.

"Cytoxan is used to treat a few different types of cancer and that does include breast cancer. The side effects include nausea or vomiting (may be severe), loss of appetite, stomach pain or upset, diarrhea, temporary hair loss (head, eyebrows, eyelashes, and anywhere else hair grows), a wound that will not heal, missed menstrual periods, changes in skin color (darkening), or changes in nails. Call me if you get pink/bloody urine, unusual decrease in the amount of urine, mouth sores, unusual tiredness/weakness, joint or bone pain, or bruising or bleeding.

"Neulasta is a bone marrow stimulant that can help the body make white blood cells after receiving the other cancer medications. You have two choices for this. You can come back to the office the day after treatment to get an injection or we can put the removable device on your arm that will dispatch twenty-five hours after treatment at home, and you can remove it or have someone else remove it after it is done dispatching. The nurses will help you understand how to do this.

"The side effects to this are bone pain, pain in your arms or legs, or injection site reactions (bruising, swelling, pain, redness, or a hard lump), fever, diarrhea, shortness of breath, rash, hair loss, numbness, nosebleeds, headache, muscle aches. Call me right away and 911 if you begin having breathing problems (e.g., trouble breathing, shortness of breath, fast breathing).

"Taxol—you won't receive this one until after you've finished the other three, so in about two-and-a-half months. Taxol is a cancer medication that interferes with the growth and spread of cancer cells in the body. It is used to treat breast cancer, ovarian cancer, and lung cancer. If you have signs of an allergic reaction to Taxol, like hives, difficulty breathing, feeling like you might pass out, swelling of your face, lips, tongue, or throat, call me and 911 immediately. If you have fever, chills, body aches, flu symptoms, sores in your mouth and throat, pale skin, feel light-headed or short of breath, rapid heart rate, trouble concentrating, easy bruising, unusual bleeding (nose, mouth, vagina, or rectum), purple or red pinpoint spots under your skin, flushing (warmth, redness, or tingly feeling), slow heart rate, feeling like you might pass out also call me and come into the office. The normal side effects are much less than the other medicines but include the potential for seizure (convulsions), chest pain, dry cough, wheezing, feeling short of breath, numbness, tingling, or burning pain in your hands or feet (also known as neuropathy), jaundice (yellowing of the skin or eyes), or severe redness or swelling, severe irritation, a hard lump, or skin changes where the injection was given. You could experience mild nausea, vomiting, diarrhea, constipation, weakness, joint or muscle pain, darkening of your skin or nails, and temporary hair loss."

The room was quiet after she went through everything, and she then asked, "Are you nervous? What's wrong?"

Immediately, I welled up with tears. "I don't know if I want to do this. What if it doesn't work? What if I can't take all this medicine? It sounds like it's going to kill me anyway!"

She put her hand on my knee, and her eyes began to water. She responded, "You have babies. You have to try everything for them. We will take good care of you. We will help you get through this. I promise."

Corey grabbed my hand and whispered, "It's okay."

Looking back as we recall this moment, he says that all he could think about was wanting to nurture me and let me know that he had my back, no matter what. I think if I had decided at that moment that I didn't want to do it, he would've politely thanked the doctor for her time, and we would have walked right out of that office. However, that's not what we decided. I dried my tears as best as I could and then looked back down at the pamphlet. Corey took my hand, and he grabbed the papers and stuffed them down into my bag.

We finished the conversation with Dr. Salem with her reassuring me, and she walked us over to the infusion room where I once again saw that nurse that had hugged me the first time we met. Dr. Salem read off my report to the nursing staff and told me to hang in there. The nurses told me to choose my seat and followed me over to the last seat in the very back of the infusion room. This would become my spot (in my best Sheldon voice of the *Big Bang Theory*).

The chair that I chose had a beautiful view of Lake St. Louis. I was also out of talking range of any of the other patients as I wasn't quite ready to be social about why I, a thirty-four-year-old young woman, was getting treated for cancer. I didn't even want to talk about it with myself. The nurses came back, super-friendly and sweet, and began putting on the armor of an old-time soldier; well, at least that's what it felt like. They were in full-length disposable gowns, gloves, and masks.

The thought immediately crossed my mind, *If you need to wear all of that to inject me, why should this be put in my body again?* The chemo medical bag from the pharmacist had the skull and crossbones, and I was sitting there with a straight face, silently losing my mind. *Well, here goes nothing!* The nurses took the time to carefully pull back the bandage that Dr. Vaughn had put on the day before. They used my newly accessed port to hook up to the IV dispenser that would begin to pour this medicine into my body. The fight with cancer officially begins. It took a full four hours for the first treatment, and they sent me home with a lovely parting gift—Neulasta. So, in twenty-five hours from the time it was attached, the medicine would be dispatched on its own, and once it was completed, I could remove it from my arm. If it were only that simple!

Chemotherapy was not easy. In fact, it was downright hard. In total, I ended up in the ER four times with one of those visits turning into a two-night stay. I had two occasions where treatment was denied due to my blood levels not being good enough, and the risk of infection being too great. Missing those sessions pushed out my desired and planned completion date for completing treatment, which made me upset and frustrated. To make matters worse, there was absolutely nothing I could have done about it. Hindsight being twenty-twenty, you realize that these delays were purposeful.

I can recall a few times through treatment where I had all but given up. I was completely miserable, showing every side effect that was listed on the side of the bottle, and sometimes fluids coming out of every exit I had! There was one breaking point where I looked at Corey straight in his eyes and told him I didn't want to continue. With tears streaming down my face, I said, "I quit! I don't want to do this anymore. I can just stop treatment. I'm tired of throwing up, I'm tired of being tired, not being able to hug my kids or hold water down. I'm tired of lying in bed and I'm tired of feeling like this. Just let me go!"

He sat quietly on the bathroom floor, staring back at me. I could tell if heartbreak could be worn on the outside, this is what it would look like. In a small voice and tears flowing down his cheeks, he let me finish and then replied, "I can't tell you how you feel and I can't even tell you to fight, but I can tell you that I need you. We need you. Baby, please...I promise we can get through it, I have you...I have you completely. I love you."

I gazed back at him, and something inside whispered, "You have to push! You have to PUSH (Pray Until Something Happens)!"

Reading through and remembering all of the side effects, the subsequent things that did happen, and the realization that I made it through was reassuring. It should be for you as well. Regardless of the situations we face, there is always an end that will occur. In the Bible, it reads:

To everything there is a season, and a time to every purpose under the heaven: A time to be born, and a time to die; a time to plant, and a time to pluck up that which is planted; a time to kill, and a time to heal; a time to break down, and a time to build up; a time to weep, and a time to laugh; a time to mourn, and a time to dance; a time to cast away stones, and a time to gather stones together; a time to embrace, and a time to refrain from embracing; a time to get, and a time to lose; a time to keep, and a time to cast away; a time to rend, and a time to sew; a time to keep silence, and a time to speak; a time to love, and a time to hate; a time of war, and a time of peace. (Ecclesiastes 3:1–8)

This passage of scripture is a confirmation that there is a beginning and an ending to every obstacle, situation, and circumstance we face in life. It may not be easy, but that is part of the pruning process, the process that we must go through to learn a lesson or several lessons, to heal, to forgive, to understand, to thrive in the life that we have been given. Or, more simply put to bloom where we are planted.

In listening, thinking, and feeling, you should also allow yourself to be vulnerable and sensitive to positive attributes to your spirit. I learned a powerful lesson from my eight-year-old son. On Sunday afternoon, I needed to take the kids to my mom's house to attend a friend's event as Corey was serving on an army drill weekend. Shortly after we entered the highway, Corey Jr. asked, "Mommy, is there another way we can take to Granny's house?"

My response was, "Yes, but it takes a little longer to go that way."

To which he responded, "Well, that's okay, right? Because we'll still get to Granny's house no matter which way we take."

I looked down at the clock and reasoned with myself. *I'm running early, he doesn't make these types of requests often, and it won't hurt for him to learn multiple ways of getting to new destinations, and he'll get a feel for new landmarks.* At the same time, I thought this may be God redirecting me to avoid an accident or a delay. So, we proceeded to merge onto a different highway and take the longer route to my mom's house. But at that moment, there was stillness and peace that came over me.

I remained quiet and listened to the dialog in the backseat between my son and his four-year-old twin sisters. He said to them, "Okay, we're going a different way, but guess what? Mommy is still taking us to Granny's house. We'll get to see some new things too!"

The girls became excited. Even though we'd taken this highway before, we'd never taken this route to Granny's house. Within a few minutes, we were crossing a bridge, and Corey Jr. instructed the girls to look over to the right out of the window. "Look over there, that's the bridge that we usually cross, but this way is new, so we have to keep our eyes open and remember we have a new way too."

It felt like a ton a bricks hit me. What I could only feel was the Holy Spirit had imparted a major lesson on my heart through the eyes, words, and faith of my children. At this juncture in my breast cancer journey, it seemed like I was experiencing delay after delay and disappointment after disappointment, but I hadn't thought of the way Corey Jr. explained. God was putting me on another route, redirecting my path, but ultimately, even if it took a little longer, I'd still arrive at the same destination. My kids had faith that even though we were taking a new route, Mommy knew how to get them where they needed to go without fail. And that tipped me further into my faith that God knew the destination and had a plan that was best for me, but I had to trust him through everything, even in those things that seemed as though "weren't going in the right direction." I had to believe that I was not on this journey for no reason and that every delay or redirection was an intercession that needed to take place for my own benefit.

I thought back to chemo when I was rejected for treatment because my blood levels and readings were too low. At the time, I was so upset. I cried because I had gotten into a routine, and I knew my date of completion would now be shifted. But now, clear as day, I saw that shift was for my benefit. I allowed my body extra time to recover. It allowed me time to be present with my husband and kids and not be sick, running back and forth to the bathroom, lying in bed or on the floor. I had extra time for my body to do some self-healing and prepare for my next treatment.

As fate would have it, two days after this request to reroute and my realization from the Holy Spirit, my cousin texted me, informing me that she had been diagnosed with cervical cancer. Here was my opportunity to encourage someone else, a life that was close to me, one that I knew I had to be the example.

Sarah Jakes Roberts, another one of my favorite ministers, explained the idea of restructuring in life. In this sermon, entitled "Restructuring," she provided timely insight of what happens and why we go through trials and tribulations of life. She leads that in order for me to walk in my anointing, I need to restructure, being intentional about the version of me that needs to live and the version of me that needs to die.

Restructuring requires me to let go of what I think I know and embrace what God is calling me to do. I have to change my mind about who I am because I can't be who I used to be and who I need to be at the same time. More and more, I'm becoming more aware, accurate, and intentional. I'm coming to a place where I can see it. I can't continue to function the way I had been functioning—out of lack, depression, fear, and anxiety. I'm called to step into the promised land.

There are things that you lose along the way that may not necessarily feel good. The greatest obstacle that we have to cover is getting out of the habit of being the underdog!

That statement reigned so true for me. It is the realization that you can't speak the Word and still see yourself the same way you've always seen yourself. Everything about you is different— the way you walk, the way you talk, the way you move and go about your day, the words you speak, and the tone you use to express your thoughts. It's all different.

Corey told me that the way I pray now is different. It's a different relationship that I have with my Father. Pastor Sarah closed her sermon with, "If he didn't take my hunger after all I've been through, that is a sure sign that it's not over. I'm just restructuring."

We have to make the choice not to give up during the restructuring. In fact, we should surrender to it, to the goodbyes and the hellos, to a new level of belief, thinking, and being. The world has a need for you. It's making new demands. On the other side of the battle, the beauty that rises from the ashes is a version of you that you didn't even know existed!

It's absolutely true that any transition or change is hard. Going through the process brought me down. I died to myself often, and then I realized that I needed to die to live. I had to continue the death, burial, and resurrection until I understood what that process meant for me. It no doubt is absolutely terrifying, not knowing, having no control, or not being able to predict what the end will be. What matters is the fight, the gift of continual perseverance and resilience that will push you into your next season. Take a break when you need to.

I was told there would be times where I just needed to let go, and letting go could mean screaming, crying, or shooting off a few rounds at the local shooting range. Whatever that looks like for you, I encourage you to feel what you feel and then allow the restructuring to continue. If you go through life always comfortable, no dreams, ambitions, or desires you have will ever come to pass. More times than not, you have to work, work hard, bruise your hands and knees, be tired and worn out, but it's for the greater good.

CaringBridge Journal Entry: The Rumble
Journal entry by Anastasia Stevenson—April 12, 2019

Long Post Alert
After each chemo session so far, the following 3–4 days I'm completely wiped out. This time it took a huge hit to my head, heart and faith. I wrestled with so many thoughts from the typical "why" to "why is this so hard" to "where are you God?" I couldn't feel Him, hear His voice and the Word was not alive to

me. My heart was broken, and I didn't know how to find my way out. This is the part that most don't tell. The behind-the-curtain of the hurt and pain, not physically, but the emotional strain body, mind, and soul.

This past week, I've cried and wet up my sister's (Zundra) shirt! I've buried my head in my husband's chest and fell completely to the floor. I've stared at my kids for hours, trying to figure out how to keep them inspired, normal, and carefree while I deal with a broken heart. *But God!* I decided to do things differently and share with a few people how I had been feeling, especially when I felt God wasn't present. The best thing I could have done...my warriors came through. Not just with words of encouragement but with Bible verses, worship songs (even some being sung *live*), and prayer coverings. Daily reminders of when God seems quiet is usually when he is waiting on me to lay it all on him...and *that* is what I did. I was honest about my feelings of being scared, fearful that my husband and kids would have to continue life without me, and scared that I'm not strong enough to carry this weight. God has been faithful and delivered to me right after I was honest with myself! I looked to find messages and books that can help me feel more normal and inspire me along the way. One of the posts I read was from Dr. Jackie Walters of Married to Medicine. Dr. Jackie is a two-time survivor. She said, "Go ahead and cry, get it out, and once you're done, let's fight, and there's no way to win a fight with tears in your eyes!" She went further and said, "When you look good, you feel good!" Those messages stirred up the fight in me. I was able to build out a positive affirmation sheet to post in my bedroom, review and re-post on my vision board, finish reading *Rising Strong* by Brene Brown (highly recommended) and begin reaching out to support groups and yoga studios that specialize in patients with cancer.

A couple of things that I am currently facing are some minor chest pains, bone and muscle pain, and some uncertainty around how the medicines are working with the tumors. I had an echo done yesterday to check my heart and will get those results on Tuesday when I see the doctor. I'm also being scheduled for another scan to check the size of the tumors and their response to the medications thus far.

I have two more rounds of chemo with the two current medications which have taken *all* of my hair, are turning my nails black, slowly decreased my ability to be in closed public spaces (due to my immune system being weak), and have wreaked havoc on my appetite. After these two sessions are complete, I'll move forward to a new medication for my final 12 rounds of chemo to complete the chemo cycle. Those cycles produce a different set of side effects. We'll cover those later!

The beautiful thing about this process is seeing and feeling the love of my family, especially my husband. Marriage is often tested under hard circumstances, and this is definitely tough! Corey has been my everything! He's picked me up off the shower floor and the toilet, he's walked me upstairs, sat in the ER room at all times of the night, helped me make critical decisions to my health, held me when I cried in the middle of the night, knowing he has to be in the office the next day, and he's the one who shaves my head! His love for me is amazing. I'm blown away by how he takes care of me! Why is it so overwhelming? Great question! Corey and I have been struggling so long to find out how to communicate and really love each other… this hard thing has brought us so close that I'm overjoyed with us and our growth.

Being able to accept the love that is being given to me has been challenging, but the growth that is already occurring is so awesome and amazing. Thank you for being on this ride with us. For your love and support. We are grateful! I've included a couple of pictures from the final shaving of my head.

Those who sow in tears shall reap in joy and singing (Psalms 126:5 AMPC)

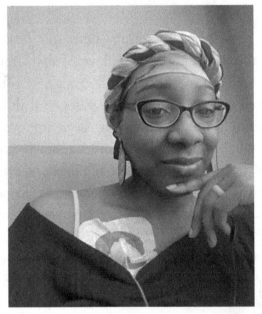

Anastasia at the chemo center during treatment.

CaringBridge Entry: The HOPE Cycle
Journal entry by Anastasia Stevenson—May 18, 2019

This morning is a tough morning… to be honest, the last two weeks have been tough. I had an expectation that after the last double dose of the first cycle medicines, things would get easier. Ha! After that cycle, I was hospitalized for a couple of days on heavy antibiotics and then released. Then, I had a break…and I started to feel better. We got ready for the fifth round, a new drug called Taxol. Well, according to studies, this medicine was supposed to be a walk in the park compared to the others. Long story short, it sucks just as bad.

Complete transparent moment, I've been in tears, throwing up, ready to give up, talking through options with Corey on whether to continue this fight this way or how I can make things "easier" on him and our family. The devil had risen up in me... I had given him space to do so. I began to give up instead of calling on the one who made me.

As I'm writing this post, I'm still nauseous, still ready to take off to the bathroom...but something told me I needed a word this morning. So I logged into Elevation Church and listened to the Mother's Day sermon given by Holly Furtick. It's called the Hope Cycle. Essentially, she displays Roman's 5:3–4, in summary: Hope—suffering—perseverance—character—*hope!* What I got from it was that in this time, I'm expected to get weak, mad, frustrated, sad, but I am not to stay there because my suffering will bring forth perseverance that builds an unshakable character that yields dividends in more Hope of who My God is and what He is able to do. She went on to say that while we ask all of those questions like why me, why now, etc., we miss the biggest question of Do I Trust God?! Do I trust Him to bring me out, that the Great work He started in me he will be faithful to complete! Whose report will I believe?!

This is by far the hardest thing I've done in my life, BUT I will Trust God. I'm not perfect, I will fall again, but I will get back up. Romans 5:3–4, "Not only so, but we[a] also glory in our sufferings, because we know that suffering produces perseverance; perseverance, character; and character, hope."

On August 6th, at approximately 11:00 a.m. CST, I rang the bell with tears in my eyes. Ringing the bell is symbolic of successfully closing the chapter to this phase of treatment and moving forward to what's next. I invited family friends to participate in my chemotherapy completion bell-ringing ceremony. It was a great turn out; even my favorite nurse brought in treats. Things, of course, did not go as planned. My treatment was behind schedule and prolonged my time at the office. Circling me were family and friends with bells of their own, ringing them loudly and proud that this chapter had been closed. There were shouts of praise, "Hallelujah and Glory" were loudly sung! I prayed silently, thanking God for bringing me through this rough part of the journey. It was only Him who had carried me this far.

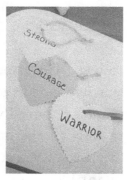

"Love Notes" handed out during treatment
that reminded me WHO I am!

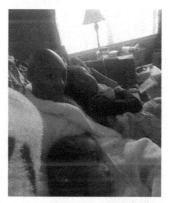

Anastasia with her two daughters, Aaliyah & Kennedi, post
treatment. Words cannot express the emotion of this moment.

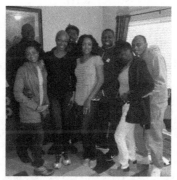

Anastasia & her husband with the Stevenson family
from Nashville, TN! It meant the world to have
them come to St. Louis to check up on us!

~Surgery~

The night before surgery, I had spent all day sweeping, mopping, vacuuming, laundering—just about anything to keep me moving. I kept my mind occupied with Amazon Prime's Beyoncé station blaring through the house—because "Who runs the world? *Girls!*" My anxiety was at an all-time high, but my outer demeanor wouldn't allow it to shine through. On the outside, I was calm, organized, and pretending to be in control. I wanted to feel I had control of me, my emotions, state of being, my mind, and my heart; yet, the internal struggle was real. I received a few texts from friends that they loved me, were thinking of me and were praying for me. It made me feel good that my support system was in full force. Yet, there was always that feeling of wishing that someone would call, and to know that they wouldn't, was heart-wrenching.

For me, the voices that I longed to hear were those of my dad and my great-grandmother. My dad passed away when I was young, twelve years old, to be exact, and in my eyes, he could do no wrong. I taught him to write his name in cursive and in print. He was my superhero. My dad spent his days just living. He had only middle school education, and my brothers and sisters (technically half brothers and sisters) and I debated about where my dad was born. We agreed on Mississippi but not the town/city, so I stuck with Meridian since it was on my birth certificate.

My dad encouraged me, defended me, and loved me with every fiber of his being. I was truly a "daddy's girl." It broke my heart when he died, and I believe he took a piece of me with him. If he were here, I imagine he would look at me and say, "Willie, you're going to be just fine. Now, get on your knees, say your prayers, and go to bed. I'll talk to you in the morning, be it God's will." I could almost hear him saying those words and felt comfort in believing that he would.

Now, Mrs. Laura J. Cain (her name alone is powerful to me), my great-grandmother, lived to be 109 years young. She spent the last ten years of her life living at home with my mom, my brother, and me. The majority of her life was spent in a small town called Mound Bayou, Mississippi. The stories she told me included the harsh reality of my ancestry. She was born on a plantation and, as she grew older, became what was known as a "house nigger." Her skin was a light brown sugar complexion, and she had beautiful hair. Part of her DNA was Native American.

She spent most of her time as a young girl working in the house of the plantation owner, taking care of children, cooking, and cleaning. She also told me stories of her delivering babies (amazing, right?). I remember a time she told me when she and her husband were not getting along well, they had a disagreement, and she took a train barefoot to Chicago, Illinois, to be with her family. Eventually, she returned home, and Mr. Bouise (pronounced Boo-ey) wooed her.

Grandma (what I called her) was a very special woman to me. She knew what she wanted and what she didn't. She lived in her own home alone until she was 100! She was strong in her words and in her faith. She never wore a pair of pants her entire life! We chatted about everything from slavery to civil rights to the correct way to make grits (which I have yet to master). She sang old hymns and prayed more than anyone I've ever met in my life. She also drank Milwaukee's Best beer and Crown Royal in the purple velvet bag every day until she left this earth!

Grandma taught me to always respect my mother and always make her proud, but she cheated when we played cards, sticking them into her apron pocket as if I didn't see her, and if I tried to confront her, she would just say, "Awe, girl, you just hush, whining because you are losing." Those memories always bring a smile to my face and my heart.

Grandma was one of the first people to ever say to me that God won't ever give me more than I can bear, and I don't believe those words ever took root. It wasn't until she passed that I understood her value in my life and even later in my teen years that I would begin to recall some of those good sayings, wisdom, and hymns where it would make sense. On the day she died, she told me she would be leaving. She said she was tired but that I needed to do good things and always be sweet. I promised I would, and later that evening, she went home to be with the Lord.

Grandma was amazing, and she still is. She's a light that shines bright, and it's her that I model myself after—hungering for God, having a little fun and an abundance of love for myself, family, and anyone else that crosses my path. She gives me strength, just knowing who she is and that her blood runs through my veins.

It's those two angels that God provided to me on earth that held me up during this moment as I sat thinking about what tomorrow would bring. I had elected to have a bilateral mastectomy—removal of all breast tissue in both my left and right breasts, even though the cancer was only on my left side. Both nipples and areolas would be removed during this surgery as well. The night prior to surgery, I ate up until the cut off as required by my doctors, nothing after midnight. I completed my special shower to prep for surgery, changed the linens on the bed, and washed with the appropriate soap. I'd spent quality time with my husband, children, and mother and did whatever I thought I could to control the environment. I rose at 5:00 a.m. for some early pillow chat with Corey. I released my concerns, my fears, and my feelings, and then I became intentional about my thoughts. It was here that I recalled, "as a man thinketh, so he is" (Proverbs 23:7). We had discussed the night before that my mom would drive me to the hospital so that Corey could drop off the kids at school, and they'd start their day as normal as possible. They all gave me sweet kisses, and I told them I'd see them later. CJ was very aware and asked a few questions. "Mom, will you have your surgery today?"

I responded, "Yes, baby, but I will be back home before you and your sisters are home from school."

I could tell he was nervous, so I hugged him tight and promised that no matter what, I'd be okay. He seemed a little relieved and then replied, "I love you, Mom."

I responded with an "I love you too, big boy," and we separated. On the way to the hospital, I was quiet and remained in conversation with my heavenly Father, making my request known to him—that he would keep me in perfect peace and take care of my family during this time.

We arrived at the hospital and did all the standard check-in procedures. They provided Corey the lingo for the board so that he'd know which place I was and could keep track of my progress during surgery. The nurse explained that this would be a longer surgery as they would be removing the breast tissue and some of the lymph nodes under my arm. The amount of lymph nodes removed would be determined by a little blue dye that would be put into the area to trace how far the cancer had spread. We discussed the implications, reviewed all the paperwork. My mom was there with me, snapping selfies of bright smiles. I had also asked one of my brothers, Howard Jr., to come back and pray over me. He did such and again confirmed that I would be fine.

We began the walk down to surgery, and the nurses showed my family where they'd sit and wait for me. She encouraged them to go grab some food and promised she'd contact them if there were any issues. Each one gave me hugs, but Corey saved his love for last. He came up to me, looked me in my eyes, and told me, "You got this." I gave him a kiss and told him I'd see him later.

In pre-op, it's the worse! You sit alone until the nurse comes back to give you premeds to help you "relax." We then get the pep talk from the surgeon, and she asks me to confirm the procedure I'm having. My glasses were moved and put in a small baggie labeled "Stevenson." All the paperwork is squared away, and then we begin to roll back to the operation room. When everything was said and done, surgery had taken a little over five hours.

~Post-Surgery~

As I awoke in the recovery room, I opened my eyes to nurses that were monitoring my stats. Everything, as I was told, had gone according to plan. There were no issues, no setbacks, nothing that jeopardized my life. Praise God! And that is the praise that was raised up on the inside of me. Corey and I had discussed upon waking up we'd have an inside joke. That joke was that when we made eye contact. I say, "Babe, I don't have no nipples!" as Kevin Hart had done in a comedy special that we had watched together a few weeks prior. It would be a moment to break the ice and also begin to embrace my new normal.

I did, in fact, do just that. However, I learned that I had not just done it with him but also with the nurse that was watching over me in recovery. By God's grace, she took no offense and also chuckled a bit herself as she too had been through the same surgery. Still in recovery, my family was allowed to come back. My husband, mom, and best friend, Brandi, were all waiting for me. As I was covered in tons of blankets and now snacking on Cheez-It crackers and Sprite, my best friend, Brandi, turned on some praise and worship. It was one of my favorite songs sung by Koryn Hawthorne entitled "Won't He Do It." She snapped pictures of me mumbling the words but hands up in total praise, knowing that God had done it. The nurses explained my drains and ensured that I could hold the food down as we began getting me ready to go home. It was done, and God had carried me through.

A little over five hours of surgery to remove over nine lymph nodes, all breast tissue, and also my nipples and areolas, I found myself contemplating all that had occurred up to this point and giving God praise. Though the parts were missing, his masterpiece was still intact. I had life to continue to live.

Comparatively, the surgery was the easiest of the first three phases. Essentially, all I had to do was not eat and go to sleep and let everyone else handle the rest! It required me to take orders and be still. I was off of work, on leave at this point, and my job was to recover. The day after surgery, I reported back to the plastic surgeon. I was sore and extremely stiff. I used the back entrance to his office, which is a lovely addition to any surgical office, and went in to see Dr. Mills.

He checked over the drains (the worst part of this surgery) and took a closer look at the incisions. This was the first time I would see my chest with no nipples or areolas. It was shocking, and I was in disbelief. I really can't explain the way I felt. It was a weird sensation of joy that the cancer no longer resided in my body but also a mourning of who I was before this whole thing began. I looked in the mirror and took a deep breath. I was still covered with pink tape in the form of a makeshift bra. The expanders were in and would stretch my skin and help me prepare for the implants that would be inserted after radiation was completed.

The weeks following would be targeted at watching my drains and ensuring they are pulling the fluid from within the wound. I would get up and out, pushing myself to the limit, having Corey to walk with me around the neighborhood to get my heart rate up, get the blood circulating, and get some good sunlight. I'd have a number of doctor appointments, which became familiar and expected. It seemed my life revolved around some type of doctor's office. I was grateful to them and their staff members. They all played a critical role in getting me through.

The time would come when the drains came out and the process to heal came to move forward with the next portion of treatment. To each ending of a phase, I raise a holy hallelujah, being grateful that God has seen me through. Faith was tested throughout the journey, but I held on. I think it was during the last few rounds of chemo when I began to see joy in ordinary things—the sun shining, the kids laughing, or just being able to clean or do laundry without assistance. I began to notice the things that I took for granted, like the ability to just move around, drive myself, and take care of our home. This temporarily removed from me helped me to see why I had every reason in the world to just be thankful; another necessary lesson learned on the road to healing.

CaringBridge Journal Entry: September 04, 2019
Journal entry by Brandi Henry—September 4, 2019

Hey, Fam!
I just wanted to give you all a quick update on Stasi. She is out of surgery and doing *so good!* We are currently in recovery and she is praying, rejoicing and singing praises to *God!* Hallelujah! #WontHeDoIt Once she is done with recovery, we will take her home to rest and recover. She will respond to your messages of love and support as soon as she is up to it. I'm sure she will make a post here as well. Until then, keep praying! They are still in need.

—Brandi

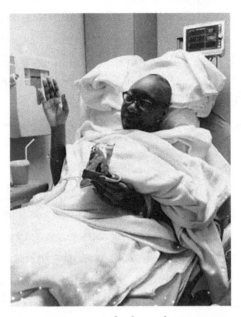

Anastasia post-surgery–bi-lateral mastectomy and placement of expanders—with a WORSHIP!

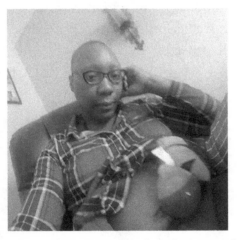

Anastasia 1 day post op with 3 drains in place

~Post-Surgery Recovery~

I went home from the hospital with three medical drains whose purpose was to remove any fluid that would accumulate during the healing process. These plastic doohickeys would go wherever I go and be the most annoying thing ever! They did well in that I had no infections and suctioned the fluids from the necessary places as they were expected to do.

During the visit, Dr. Mills said we would not do any manipulation, but I would see him in about a week to begin the inflation process. The goal at this point was to monitor the output of the drains and ensure the amount was decreasing. The magic number was 30 ccs. Once the fluid decreased to 30ccs, the drains would be removed. That's what I needed, something to work toward, a goal that would tell me that good progress was being made and that my body would find its way back to a somewhat normal state of being.

In the process of getting this news, I also received another phone call from a "breastie" also known as a powerful woman who survived breast cancer and turned her pain into passion. Her name is Chantelle. Chantelle is the founder and CEO of an organization called The Pink Angels Foundation. She founded this organization after she was diagnosed with breast cancer, choosing to become an advocate and Wonder Woman that provided support and resources to women that were in the same battle. When Chantelle called me, September 6, she was calling to check in on my progress post-surgery and to see if I needed anything. I thought this was super-sweet as we had only met a couple of months prior, and she had been a Godsend of encouragement and inspiration to me.

Not only was she a *boss*, a loving mom, and survivor, but she had also been through the battle with close family, inclusive of her mom, an aunt, and several cousins. Through it all, she was and is positive, a trendsetter, goal-oriented, and an amazing friend. This phone call didn't end with pleasantries, though. She asked how I would feel about walking the field with her on September 14 at the St. Louis Cardinals game and throwing out the first pitch. My mouth flung open, and I said yes, not even giving a second thought to having just had a pretty major surgery. This would be less than a week away. But here is also where my brain and my body disconnected. What I thought I heard her say was "walking with me and standing with me while I went through the pitch," but what she had actually said was, "Join me, and you throw the pitch." Potato, po-tah-to, right?

I told Corey all about it, and he said, "Cool, let's make it a family thing. We'll get the kids and take a stroll around and get you back home, but we have to be careful. You still have drains in, and we don't want any type of problems."

"I promise I'll be on top of it. Have my pain meds ready to go, and if need be, we'll leave whenever the moment strikes us."

Fast-forward, we get to the stadium. It's Sista Strut weekend. Sista Strut is a nonprofit focused on bringing breast cancer awareness to the African American community. It's celebrated with a parade and tons of festivities throughout the city.

We go about our Saturday, get the kids ready to go, meet up with some friends and family, and then Chantelle and I take a walk with the infamous BJ the DJ down to the "First Pitch" room. I had no idea about this part of the stadium where the business happens and all the behind the scenes action is going on. We were scanned and escorted in with a larger group. I also learned this day that there were multiple first pitches! Seriously,

I had no clue! So we all got lined up and ready to go. I met some wonderful people, including the GM of the St. Louis Cardinals, the sponsor of the main stage supporting Sista Strut, Prophetess Nona M. Thomas, and some phenomenal lawyers from the Brown and Crouppen law firm! It was amazing!

I was standing on the field of the St. Louis Cardinals, and then I turned to Chantelle and said, "Okay, here you go."

Her response was, "No, you're throwing it!"

What! I was super-thrilled, honored, and blown away that she'd asked me to be part of this, but I got to throw the pitch! Heck, *yeah!* Drains and all, we had to make this happen. We had done a good job that morning securing the drains to a camisole underneath my shirt, which was also underneath the Pink Angels jersey that I was wearing in support of the organization. After six other first pitches, it was our turn. I turned to Fred Bird who was ecstatically ready to escort me out onto the pitcher's mound, but I wasn't ready. I had butterflies for days, and there were people in those seats…thousands of people, and amongst those people, my husband, three children, brother and sister-in-law, cousins, and a host of great friends showing their support. But the time was now.

Suddenly, I didn't feel any pain, no discomfort, but I wasn't completely crazy either. Fred Bird told me to go where I was comfortable and go for it. And before I knew it, *the pitch was good! Straight over home plate!* My arms went straight up in the air, and Cardinals Pitcher John Tyler Webb (#30) caught my ball! I am still in awe of that moment. I hugged Chantelle, the prophetess, and Fred Bird tightly, and with a smile like no other, began walking back to my seat! Still in awe, I shook BJ the DJ's hand and thanked him for the opportunity. Can we say Cloud 9? I was sailing! I don't remember walking back to my seat, but I do remember the girls spotting me and telling me over and over that they saw me on the big screen and they saw me throw the ball, and we saw FRED BIRD! How amazing was that!

Shortly thereafter, the adrenaline was leaving, and I could no longer fake my pain. I tapped Corey and told him it was time to go. He wasted no time. I hugged Chantelle bye and told her that I would never forget this moment, and I thanked her for choosing me. Funny things began to happen, though, as we began to walk out. Women I had never seen before stopped me. They told me that just doing that, throwing the ball, gave them hope, inspiration, and strength. *Wow*, I wasn't expecting that at all! I looked at these women individually, and the pain that I felt seemed necessary. It was necessary that they see someone going through what they were going through who was smiling and still deciding to live.

One young lady cried, and before I knew it, I grabbed her in my arms and told her that this too would pass and she was never fighting alone. She felt my drains and looked me in my eyes. My response was, "See, you just never know. If I can do this, you most certainly can."

Corey only allowed this to happen twice more as he could see the pain in my face. We took an elevator down, and I waited with security while he brought the car around.

What I know to be true is when you are at the peak of what feels like happiness, there comes some stumbling block to try to knock the wind out of your sails. In the birth of these moments, I had to write down the feelings that had become apparent inside of me, words that were formed through a dream of a loved one that had won the ultimate battle. He had gone to Jesus after a tough battle with cancer. I am choosing not to reveal his name as I know there are pains that are still being processed around his untimely departure from our home to his heavenly home.

In this dream, I chased him. I pursued his presence because there was something that I knew he would be able to reveal to me through this process. The process of death, though this may not have been my path, I knew, ultimately, I would need to walk along the road; and with a diagnosis like cancer, the final say could be now, or it could be much later. So, in this dream, I chased after him. I ran through long hallways with hopes of him turning around and giving a nod of "I'm okay" or "It isn't that bad." But I couldn't quite reach him. It seemed the harder I ran, the further he moved from me.

Finally, in a place toward the top of what seemed like a huge hill, he turned toward me, and with him, standing on his right, was a presence of what had to be God. There was no face that I could see, no building or structure that I could go into detail about, but a significant presence that left me both speechless and in awe. So much so that my only desire was to fall to my knees and begin what could be described as fervent prayer or complete and utter surrender of my own thoughts, desires, or anything that could have captured or distracted me from this moment.

As I looked at my loved one, his face displayed happiness, joy, peace, and love. He had no trace of the battle he'd been through, no scars or imperfections, no pain or unsettlement but victory and gladness. At this moment, with that last image, I sat straight up in bed. I reached for my husband in full tears. Deep moans and cries welled up from my belly, and I searched for a notebook. I searched for a pen because I had to write this down. Here was the answer that I had been seeking, the understanding that I believed I needed. So, on September 23, 2019, at approximately 4:45 a.m., I wrote the following:

> **Stop Running**. I've got you. In the presence of the Lord, there is nothing to do but bow and worship. The Spirit takes over and provides confirmation of peace, joy, and love. Nothing is wasted, and there is everything to gain. God is love. Cancer is my vehicle to see him face-to-face. Be strong and courageous in the belief that there is nothing to fear— God has you. A spiritual encounter with a loved one that has passed away, is with him, and his love is in abundance. They are happy, healthy, and whole in the presence of God. I fellowship in joy, peace, love, and surrender. Standing in the light that streams high and bright.

Reflecting on this moment and the time that it was written, I was a few weeks past my bilateral mastectomy and had been feeling a lack of identity of who I was and afraid of who I may never become. I had for so long put trust in "stuff" and not in the one that created me, knitted me in my mother's womb, and knew everything that I would face before even taking my first breath. It was an emotional state of being. Nothing was the same, and yet, there was so much more to learn about possibilities and the opportunities that God provided to be within his peaceful dwelling of living life through a different lens. We see and feel pain from a loved one passing, but that is the human way. If we push a little differently, squint our eyes to reveal a different perspective, choose to seek God's truth, we will live in a supernatural experience.

> CaringBridge Journal Entry: September 19, 2019
> Journal entry by Anastasia Stevenson—September 19, 2019

Hi, Family,

I hope this note finds you all happy, healthy, and whole!

I'm sorry for the delay in posting an update, but the healing process is real...physically and mentally! Since my last update, I'm up moving around, taking walks, and I am able to dress myself...all major hurdles! Today was my third post-op visit. I won't need to see the breast surgeon for six months! That means I'm officially cancer-free! Right now, I'm scheduled to see my oncologist next week, and I'll find out what medicine I'll be assigned for the next ten years. I'll also be given a schedule to see her to maintain treatment. My port will remain in for the next year. As to the rebuilding process, I saw my plastic surgeon today. Two of the three drains have been removed. We also began pumping up the girls. I'm taking a trial run at this size and will determine if I want to hold steady or keep going next week. I'm also scheduled to see the radiologist next week. That will be moving into Phase 3! Only one more gate to go after that.

During this season, I've been provided lots of fantastic opportunities. I will be an official breast cancer support Advocate with the Pink Angels Foundation. I also had an opportunity to throw out the 1st pitch at the Cardinals game last weekend, which was so awesome! I've spent some time starting on my book, *The Evolution of Me*, and started tinkering with building my website...more information to come on both of those.

My goal is to step into God's purpose for my life and give Him the glory. God has been showing out in this process. I'm learning about God and about myself. As promised, I'm attaching two of the photos from my breast cancer photoshoot. It was an amazing experience. Thanks to my bestie, Brandi, for my makeup and setting the mood with the right tunes!

If you haven't done so already, please take some time to do your self-breast exam! I'll leave you with James 4:2 NIV: *"You desire but do not have, so you kill. You covet but you cannot get what you want, so you quarrel and fight. You do not have because you do not ask God."*

I love you!

Signed: A Survivor!

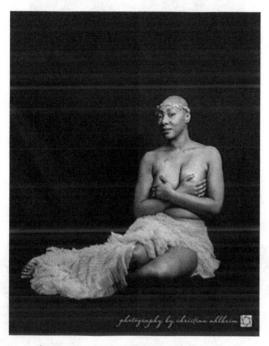

Anastasia during at home "Survivor" portrait session.
Photographer: Christina Ahlheim of Charisma Photography

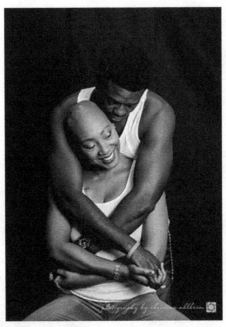

Anastasia & Corey during at home "Survivor" portrait session.
Photographer: Christina Ahlheim of Charisma Photography

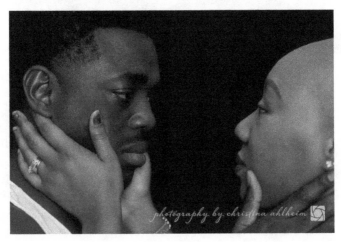

Anastasia & Corey during at home "Survivor" portrait session.
This session got really emotional.
Photographer: Christina Ahlheim of Charisma Photography

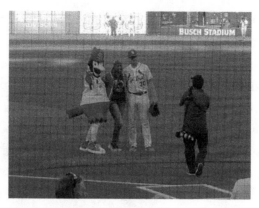

Fun with Fred Bird! Throwing out the 1st pitch
at the Cardinals game. Go CARDS! I had 3
drains pinned down underneath my shirt.

~Radiation~

The process of working to get started with radiation would begin on October eighth. I would go in for preliminary dialog about the process and understand everything that would take place. The receptionist told me to expect this to be a long appointment as there would be much work that would need to be completed in order to actually begin the radiation process. This is what I wished someone would have told me.

In preparation for radiation, several things needed to occur. I needed to be fitted properly for plastic mold that will be used for each radiation session. This mold ensures that you are lying in the same position each session, as well as be a barrier that "tricked" the laser to pushing a higher amount of radiation into my body. I also learned there was a requirement of being "tattooed." There were, in my case, five small dot tattoos placed on my skin with a small hot needle that would assist the technicians in lining up the lasers along my body, again ensuring that the same spots would receive treatment each time.

The plastic acted as skin and therefore provided the treatment area more radiation in an effort to ensure all abnormal cells were killed. The last part was the most difficult for me, the breathing method. There was a specific method of breathing that was required during radiation to prevent the radiation beams from impacting internal organs such as the lungs and heart and all of the surrounding organs necessary to *live!* Yes, it freaked me out too! The breathing method is called Deep Inspiration Breath Hold or DIBH for short. The gist of this method is to be able to take in a deep breath, isolating the chest. You must be able to hold your breath between sixty and 120 seconds. Go ahead, give it a try. Hold your breath for an entire minute! If you are a swimmer, deep-sea diver, or anything of the sort, your timing doesn't count. But if you are not, this is a difficult task, and a frustrating one, as obtaining treatment is completely dependent on mastering this technique or at least getting good enough that treatment can take place.

In addition to those frustrations, I had to hold my arm in position for the duration of treatment, which was difficult as I had lost mobility in my left arm post the removal of the lymph nodes. This was indeed painful. I spent three sessions trying to get this right, and on the third one, I broke out in tears. I cried because I could not do it. I cried because treatment was continuing to be delayed, and I cried because it was my prerogative. I needed to let out the frustration.

I was soon thereafter, instructed that I would need to have the saline removed from the right breast expander that had been placed as a method of stretching the skin and readying my body for breast implants. This recommendation was made because of the angle of the radiation beam. If aimed directly, the beam of radiation would damage my heart, and there would be serious consequences behind that. My radiation oncologist called my plastic surgeon, and the appointment was scheduled to have the saline removed.

Upon getting to the plastic surgeon, he explained the what and the why, and we agreed it was the right thing to do. However, I was torn because this would mean that one side of my chest would be completely flat. There is absolutely no way to conceal a flat chest, or so I thought, but at that moment, it felt detrimental to my physical and mental well-being. *How will my husband react to this change? We have already changed so much. How will my kids feel if they see this "deformity" in my body? And should I explain it to them? How do I really feel about this? And am I being too damn vain for my own good?*

At the end of the day, it didn't matter. My medical team and family were behind anything that would sustain my life and give me a better chance of surviving this thing. So, I laid back on the table, and saline was removed from my right breast expander, leaving it almost flat. Once the doctor confirmed that would be enough, he assured me that after radiation was complete to call him and he'd get me right in to have the saline put back in. I told him okay and kept a straight face. The nurse provided me with some gauze to stuff my bra and give a semi-symmetrical look. Once she left, my friend and God-given sister looked at me and asked if I was okay. With only a small pause, I looked her in her eyes and replied, "No." Tears began to fall, and she wrapped me in her arms and allowed me to get it out. There was no judgment, no "but look at the bright side;" only love, protection, whispered prayers for strength, and the awesome power of a healing touch.

I pulled myself together, and without pause, Zundra said, "Now's a good time to go shopping for the girls. Let's take our minds off this and have some fun." The girls had begun to show a growth spurt, and with everything that was going on, I had not made time to take care of this. Zundra, being who she is, jumped right in! We had a great time picking out clothes, some the same, some with variations but similar, and some things very different. But it wasn't the shopping that made me feel better. It was the genuine care that Zundra had for me. She was tough and tender and, by example, led the way for me to be the same.

After the shopping was complete, Zundra brought me back home. She came in, and together we took everything out of bags, hung clothes, put away tights, socks, and underwear and laughed *a lot!* It was a therapy session that I needed, one on one! After she left, I journaled a bit and then focused. I lay on the floor, Googled some YouTube videos on DIBH, and decided when I went back to radiation, I would have mastered this technique and would receive treatment.

Once Corey got home that evening, I solicited his help. His job was to tell me when to take my deep breaths, ensure that no other parts of my body moved while taking these breaths, and then time me. He was more than happy to help me master this and had complete confidence that I would be able to rock this out. The first two tries were unsuccessful, but then he looked me in my eyes and whispered, "You got this, you can do this." And I believed him.

The next try was good. I stayed in position, isolated my body, and held my breath for sixty seconds! That was good but I needed it to be better, just in case the treatment hit that eighty-second timeline. We continued to practice, and I got better and better. The seconds were adding up, and I began knowing when my body was about to expire and redirected my thoughts by encouraging my inner fighter. "You got this, Stacy, hold it!"

As God would have it, at my next appointment with the radiation team, there was a specialist in the building. The night prior, the hospital system had an upgrade, and it required a specialist on-site to ensure the staff was trained, the technicians knew best practices, and the patients had a better experience. This specialist happened to also have been a DIBH expert. With so much joy and excitement, my technician came out to get me set up and try to get the placement correct for the films that were required before treatment. They introduced me to the specialist and told me she was one of the best, and if anyone could get me going, it would be her.

Per the instructions, I took my first deep breath and began to hold as Corey and I had practiced, and immediately, the specialist said, "Wait, no, let it out." She asked, "Have you ever danced or done gymnastics?"

It was an odd question, but my answer was yes! I had studied dance (ballet, tap, jazz, hip-hop, and modern) as a child and danced through adulthood.

She exclaimed, "*That's it!* Forget about your posture and holding in your stomach as you were taught when you danced. Think only about the rising of your chest and the expanding of your belly. With that simple direction, my next DIBH was perfect! *The best feeling ever!* That small tweak shifted everything!

The techs stepped out of the room and began taking films. I watched as the machine moved around me, listening to the clicks, bangs, and bongs. And then over the loudspeaker, the tech said, "We're almost done! Just a few more minutes, Stacy, and we'll be right in."

A couple of clicks and bongs later, the ladies walk back into the room. I asked, "Can we start treatment now?"

And the response was, "You just finished your first treatment!"

Can we say praise break? I had completed my first radiation treatment and didn't have a clue! What a rewarding moment! I thanked the specialist over and over and hugged my technicians so tight. I would be seeing them every day now, Monday through Friday, to receive my radiation treatments, twenty-eight in total.

Around the fourth week of radiation, my skin started to change. This is what is called burning from radiation beam. I essentially was being cooked from the inside out. I chose not to shift from schedule because I had a desire to be done with radiation before Thanksgiving so that we could get this all closed out in 2019. The technicians were kind enough to work a Sunday for me and several other patients that had the same request. That last session, my skin was burned, almost crispy. It had begun to peel, and it was painful. I kept it moisturized with the recommended ointments and even added a few natural ointments of my own.

Underneath my breast, I had begun to develop an open wound where the outer layer of skin came off, and it was raw and pink. I declined wearing bras at this point and had embraced my lopsidedness. I didn't care what people thought when they saw me. They had no idea of the battle I was fighting. Then came Wednesday, November 27, my last radiation treatment. Corey and Zundra joined me at this appointment because I found out on the last treatment day, I got to ring another bell.

I prepared for treatment as I had always done but was emotional that I had made it this far. One of my favorite breasties, another breast cancer patient, Pat, was there. She hugged me so tightly and told me how proud of me she was. I didn't know Pat well, only chatted with her and her husband before and after treatments. She was sweet, kind, and she always encouraged me. People like that are a rare find. So, as I went in the radiation room and disrobed, the techs decided that we wouldn't use the plastic mode for this session due to it being the last one and that my skin had taken a pretty bad beating.

We completed treatment, and tears of happiness began to fall. I'd done it, conquered another portion of this battle. We called my mom via a mobile app as she was out of town and wanted to be part of the bell ringing ceremony. I rang the bell, and tears fell from everyone that was in the room. We'd done it. All of us! At the conclusion, they handed me a certificate that had been signed by all of my technicians and doctor that read:

Completion of Radiation Treatments

Today as you ring this bell,
It signals the close of one chapter and start of another.
Ring once for all you've endured.
Ring twice to celebrate today.
And ring once more for the future!
November 27, 2019
Congratulations to Anastasia Stevenson!
Your treatments are done,
Your course is run,
And you're on your way!

No matter how many times I read that certificate, I still get emotional. Every part of the journey had been a fight, and yet, I had not taken the time to really celebrate the steps that I'd taken to continue to move forward. It all mattered. I couldn't move forward without first completing the task at hand. It was a powerful lesson that I take with me every single day.

CaringBridge Journal Entry: Radiation Update
Journal entry by Anastasia Stevenson—November 7, 2019

Hi, Family,

I hope this note finds you happy, healthy, and whole!

Time is continuing to move and the proof is in the change of the weather. Sometimes I find it hard to believe that we've been on this journey since February of this year but that is absolutely the case!

I'm beginning to feel the effects of the radiation. I'm more tired than I've ever been. My chest is constantly tightening and I feel restricted. I'm also in a lot of pain from the expanders. From what I've read and been told, the expanders are much harder than implants and tend to hurt more when my skin is tightened around it (this is absolutely my experience). I've almost mastered that breathing technique so treatments are getting completed quicker, though holding your breath for a little over a minute is no easy task. Wednesdays are usually the longer days, as they conduct CT scans to check for damage and any potential issues, they check the penetration level of the beam to ensure it's still hitting where we need it to and providing the right amount of radiation. I also have a visit with Dr. Fu to check my skin and my mental health. We have sixteen more treatments to complete and this phase will be over. I'm being considered to be on a short list of candidates to potentially get treatment the Sunday before Thanksgiving, which will take a treatment off the back-end and get me to my goal of completion before Thanksgiving.

The next steps are to meet with Dr. Salem (chemo oncologist) to discuss when I will begin my hormone/cancer fighter pills and potential discussion of conducting a partial or complete hysterectomy. I will be on pill therapy for five to ten years. I will also meet with Dr. Mills (plastic surgeon) to re-expand the right breast and schedule the surgery to swap out the expanders for the implants... In other words, we're in the final hard stretch with a ten-year probationary period. Both appointments are in the books!

Quick story before I close out. As I was leaving radiation yesterday, another patient, Pat, and her husband asked me if they could tell me something. She said, "Whenever I see you, you greet me with a smile no matter if it's before radiation or after." She went on to say tell me that I inspire her and that she is encouraged by me because of the grace and strength she sees. She said that she didn't know what she'd do if she had to go through this with small kids and a husband in the military (her husband just happened to have retired from the army). We hugged and went our separate ways. Following this I went home, looked at my calendar to realize I had scheduled a meeting with a mentee and she was bringing two friends with her. Here is where I figured out that when I really don't want to do something is when I need to do it most. I showed up, fully present and ready for whatever they threw at me. I met with the three young, ambitious, and ready students who wanted to know what they should be doing and how to do it...to which I responded I need more information. We spent a little over two hours together... They asked questions, I answered, but what I loved most was speaking life and declaring God's Word over them. They laughed, they cried, and I encouraged both. They left with homework assignments and all three of them told me I gave them hope! We hugged and I sent them away with their heads held high and a new perspective on each of their situations. In a season that is so difficult for me, I wanted them to know that God is real and nothing is too hard for Him. As much as I wanted to cancel, I'm glad I pressed because they needed a word and I happened to be that vessel. I'm excited to see what they will do.

In closing, even though we have good and bad days, we need to know God didn't bring us this far to leave and I know he never has and never will forsake us. In the times where I struggle to want to get out of bed, to want to write, to want to do anything, I press onward and it usually pays off. What a remarkable testament of God's grace. On a day where I felt less than, weak and sad— God still shined through. It showed me, there is always someone watching and you never know how you will impact their life. So smile!

I heard this song on the radio and want to share the chorus lyrics with you. It's called "Symphony" by Switch.

'Cause even in the madness,
there is peace
Drowning out the voices
all around me
Through all of this chaos
You were writing a symphony,
a symphony'

He gives power to the faint; and to them that have no might he increases strength. (Isaiah 40:29)

I love you!

CaringBridge Journal Entry: Happy Thanksgiving
Journal entry by Anastasia Stevenson—November 29, 2019

Hi, family!

I hope this note finds you happy, healthy, whole and full of the Thanksgiving spirit!

I'm happy to report that I have completed twenty-eight rounds of radiation treatment. I cannot express how happy I am to be past this phase. Unfortunately, I did burn pretty badly so I'm dealing with trying to nurse my skin back to health and push through the pain. I was able to successfully make a carrot cake and cheesecake for the holiday and follow the instructions my mom left me to make the dressing and chitterlings. We ate as a family and spent the day with my brother and sister in love. Very low key and intimate.

This morning, I made breakfast for the kids and am now watching them put up the Christmas tree with Corey. It's quite a sight to see. I'm blessed to be here, blessed to be and feel love and blessed to be a blessing.

Over the past week or so I've watched Harriet and Frozen two. Those movies brought about the thoughts that now is the time to take the next step, to do the next right

thing and remember where you come from…
whatever that means for you.

Enjoy your families and live your best
lives! With love!

Anastasia

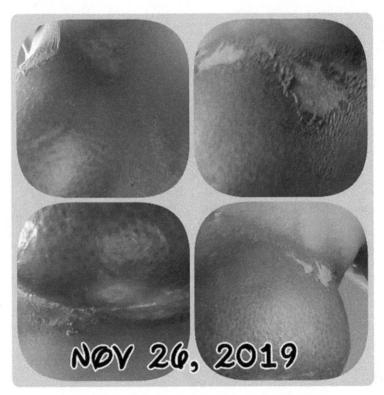

Anastasia shows her radiation burn the day before
her final radiation treatment. So super painful

Chapter 5

It's About More Than Me

And the God of all grace, who called you to
his eternal glory in Christ, after you have suf-
fered a little while, will himself restore you
and make you strong, firm and steadfast.
—1 Peter 5:10 (ESV)

Trust the process. I'm not certain who coined this state-
ment, but it is one that has proven to be more than accu-
rate. Going through the process requires identifying a plan,
creating the tasks, executing the steps, and reviewing the out-
comes. This is translated across business, personal, parenting,
coaching, surviving, and even dying. As harsh as that sounds,
it's the absolute truth.

Through this process, the process of getting rid of the can-
cer, I had to die to live. Chemotherapy drugs are formed to kill

something inside of you. Radiation is done to kill something inside of you. Surgery is performed to remove something from within you, and once that thing is on the outside, it, too, dies. The process of breast cancer brought forth the idea that in order to live, I must die. If you are a Bible reader, it is in alignment with the Word of God. It reads in Galatians 2:20, "I have been crucified with Christ. It is no longer I who live, but Christ who lives in me. And the life I now live in the flesh I live by faith in the Son of God, who loved me and gave himself for me."

This is every day you renew yourself, making yourself available to God by dying to yourself in order to be filled with the love, mercy, grace, and abundance that is rightfully yours.

Every diagnosis is different, every hormone and cell is different, but the reality we face is the same. Every woman I've had the privilege to chat with on this journey has a story that has many different variables, some that I wondered how they got through and some that I thought, *Wow, she was incredibly blessed*. But the common thread was that we all made a decision to fight, to be warriors, to go through the process and be better on the other side. Those women are happy and healthy.

In the beginning, I was angry with women who were blessed enough to have caught it early enough that no major intervention was required. I was sad that I didn't have that story. Why didn't I have that story? My journey required more invasiveness, more downtown, more pain, just more. But then my reality was jerked when I spoke to women on their second or third diagnosis, some that would have chemo for the rest of their lives, and some that would not survive the fight.

I was broken in so many ways that I couldn't see straight, but I masked that pain by pretending that my new normal would suffice because it could always be worse. I pushed myself to be involved, to go when I didn't feel like going, to talk when I didn't feel like talking, but the conversations, I ensured, would never be focused on me or my feelings. It wasn't until I was asked to consider becoming an ambassador for The Pink Angels Foundation that I would understand and come to grips with the process and my journey being individual and separate from what any other survivor went through.

As I began attending group sessions, I learned that one woman went through over forty rounds of radiation total, and another was pregnant at the time of diagnosis and still was required to undergo chemotherapy treatment. There was another woman that went through her journey completely alone because she chose not to burden her family or want to scare them. Powerful, right? Collectively, we were all amazing, intelligent mothers, daughters, wives, sisters, aunts, grand-mothers, working women, entrepreneurs, and stars in our own right with the common mission to live on purpose. The sto-ries were different, the treatments were different, the responses were different, but we were going through the same process and learning lessons from each other on how to not just survive but thrive, to shift into purpose, and to allow ourselves the right to feel whatever we needed to feel—good, bad, or ugly.

It was in this place where I began to frame a new story in my mind. I would not be afraid of what this did to me, and I would not allow it to take control of how I lived my life, and I would certainly not allow it to spark fear that could only speed up whether I lived or if I died. The story became "Here is my change and my chance." I would choose to educate others, show my battle scars, be proud of my courageousness, and empower others to make the decision to shift in spite of what the statis-tics said. I would communicate the importance that self-care also means self-checks and knowing your family history is not only necessary but a requirement; that tough conversations are necessary, and they should not be delayed because of discomfort or because "we never talk about that type of stuff." It would be time for me to step outside of myself, my fears and apprehensions to look at the bigger picture and see that it was about way more than just me.

This epiphany happened, and a bunch of other things happened too that would attempt to deter me from moving forward with a vision that I thought should be executed sooner rather than later. Once I went into praise and prayer, things seemingly started to fall apart and distracted me from the vision. The kids were going wild at school, being disrespectful, and getting into trouble. Corey and I began arguing again and not really speaking from the heart but out of exhaustion and frustration. I was disappointed with the level of support I had. It felt like people started leaving me on this journey alone, when in actuality, I had stopped communicating to them what I needed from them!

We started having issues with the house, and Christmas was coming, but our finances were low. I started to feel bad that I had invested in a company to help me write this book and I wasn't writing, so I thought it was money wasted! The struggle was so real! I was seemingly always angry, bitter, or sad. I stopped talking and shut down. But then I hit my reset button. It was about this time that I would be back in the plastic surgeon's office to talk about scheduling the final surgery to replace the expanders with silicone implants and possibly removing my port, if it would be okay with my medical oncologist.

Disappointed that the surgery would not happen in 2019, I took that as a sign that I still had some self-work to do and potentially attempt to find a way to get back to the place where

I knew I needed to be, but what was I really going to do to make this shift? I had time and opportunity. I wasn't due back to my full-time job for a while. As God would align, the founder of The Pink Angels, Chantelle, reached out to me and asked if I would be interested in applying to become a part of the Young Women's MBC (Metastatic Breast Cancer) Disparities ANGEL (Advocate Now to Grow, Empower, and Lead) Advocate Program through the Tigerlily Foundation. I told her I'd look into it and let her know. She thought it would be a great opportunity for me to learn and continue to grow and also be more well-rounded and knowledgeable in the breast cancer space.

After completing my due diligence, I talked it over with Corey, and he agreed that I should at least apply. I did, and a couple of weeks later, I was notified that I was accepted as an advocate and that I would be traveling in the coming weeks to San Antonio, Texas, to meet the other twenty-one selected advocates and attend the Annual San Antonio Breast Cancer Symposium. This trip would cost me nothing. As an advocate, the flight, hotel, and symposium fees would all be paid by Tigerlily. This would be a three-day conference, and in my mind, an opportunity for me to get a jump on the book and determine how I could best be of service to this organization. I had no idea what was in store for me.

I arrived in San Antonio and managed to navigate to my hotel, check-in, and then head down for the welcome reception. As I walked into the room full of beautiful black women, all of whom had some impact of breast cancer, I obtained my name tag and sat down for a word from the founder, Miamah Karmo, who herself was a breast cancer survivor. Miamah was passionate about hope, cures, and making it known that we, as black women, faced much worse fates in the survival of breast cancer diagnosis than any other ethnic group. I learned further that the women that had been selected to be in this group came from the most disparate cities where breast cancer killed more than 40 percent of those black women diagnosed with the disease due to lack of knowledge, lack of care, lack of basic support, and lack of access.

My heart pumped a little harder. After Miamah spoke, we went around the room and gave introductions—our names, where we were from, diagnoses, and anything else we'd like to share. Once again, I began counting my blessings. The majority of women in this room were metastatic patients. In other words, stage 4 breast cancer that had spread to organs, bones, and even the brain. Some had been diagnosed multiple times, some as early as the age of sixteen. Talk about reigniting a fire.

We would have a jammed packed schedule over the next few days but all about learning, networking, growing, contributing, and empowering against this beast called cancer. I would hear from doctors, future doctors, patients, advocates, survivors, and widowers—a humbling and necessary experience. As the days continued and I began bonding with these women, listening to their stories, I knew the calling had been confirmed. It was time to understand and dig deep on evolving through the hurt, pushing past the pain, and pursuing the purpose.

I would like to say it all happened at once, that it was quickening in my spirit, and all the pieces fell into place, but that wasn't the case. I had to go through a process of feeling, really feeling everything that I had gone through, rethinking every testimony that I'd received, and reliving moments that I'd had almost completely blocked from my mind over the past ten months.

San Antonio was a chance to dig and dig deep. While I knew that my mission there was to learn about the process of becoming an ANGEL advocate, I also knew that this was the time God had given me to rest in him, remember where I'd come from and how my story could have ended in so many different ways. San Antonio offered me a renewal of some sort. The women I'd meet and the stories I heard all brought me a surreal awakening that I didn't know I needed. It was also here in this moment that God spoke to me and told me to work with CJ to create, write, and publish *Mommy Has Cancer*. The world needed his voice too.

Returning home with a new responsibility, sense of purpose, and renewed feelings of hope and love, I returned with just enough time to go see my babies, Kennedi and Aaliyah, on stage for their Christmas show at school. My mom had done her best to dress them in the outfits I had in my head and then texted her. She put them together, and my heart was full. Corey met me at the airport and did his best to speed me out to the school where the Christmas show would be held. He was all ears and wanted to know about my experience and what had happened. His immediate question was, "What was up with the text?"

I explained that one of the sessions that I attended included a widower with two daughters. His wife had fought a good fight and went home to live in glory. He gave a powerful testimony of what he endured as a caretaker, the tough decisions he had to make, and now life without his wife and with his two little girls. It struck a chord. My heartbeat slowed, and all I could think about was Corey and all he'd been through with me. He carried so much of the battle, even though I was the one with the diagnosis.

The battle I carried, so many more fought with me. They are often forgotten or even disregarded, but they are essential in the fight for our lives. I love the mantra that no one fights alone. Even when we feel alone and isolated, like no one in the world understands the pain and suffering that we are enduring, we have to remember that we are never alone. Our loved ones, though they may not be at our fingertips, are fighting with us. They are impacted and affected. Our good friends, though they may not call every day, are affected. And our sister survivors and warriors in the fight get it!

I made the mistake of not calling on those people when I needed to the most, mainly because I felt like they all viewed me as so strong that I didn't want to appear weak. There were also times when I felt like I didn't want to be a bother or make anyone feel down or depressed, just because I was going through this thing. A close friend told me that I inspired her. She called me her "Shero." I asked her why that was. Why did she feel that way? She responded that I allowed her in. I let her see that even though this situation had me against the ropes, I never let it knock me down, and even if I went down, I came back up swinging.

It was then that I learned that people were indeed fighting for me. They were praying for me and encouraging me silently in their prayers, thoughts, and hearts. The impact that cancer had was in no way small. It reverberated through every household of every person I loved and that loved me.

Evolution hardly ever occurs in a span of seconds or minutes. It takes a while, even a period of time, to get into a space to make the decision to grow and then be determined to understand what "next" actually looks like. The key for me was to be open, to listen, to take in, to embrace, and to feel but to never stay in any of those places too long. Being there breeds negativity and lack. Lack is the last thing you need when so much has already been stripped away on the road to healing.

> As best said by Former First Lady of the United States, "For me, becoming isn't about arriving somewhere or achieving a certain aim. I see it instead as forward motion, a means of evolving, a way to reach continuously toward a better self. The journey doesn't end."
> —Michelle Obama, *Becoming*

Chapter 6

The Bonds of Sisterhood

If either of them falls down, one can help
the other up. But pity the one who falls
and has no one to help them up.
—*Ecclesiastes 4:10 (ESV)*

I realized the power of a village extremely early in my diagnosis. I didn't know how critical they would become along the journey, though. I have been blessed to meet and love many friends, associates, and then some friends that became family. Once Corey and I decided we wanted to begin to include others on the news of my diagnosis, we started slowly by telling immediate family. We knew that going this route would be easier as the word would travel fast, and people would be "in the know" without us necessarily having to individually call and talk through the pain of this over and over again. That is exactly what happened. We told a few, and very soon, after the entire family was aware. Additionally, we knew we wanted a few close friends to be included, especially since some of those friends are who we often call on in times of emergencies, like, "Can you watch the kids for date nights?" Those folks that I trust with our little people.

There were some people that I told where I felt obligation, and the response I received confirmed only distance in the relationship. It was like I could immediately tell who would be a silent supporter and who would be in the trenches with me. The reality of that stung a bit, and I learned the lesson of creating and then releasing people from the expectations I had for them in my life. Having expectations for others will either leave you over the moon happy or horribly down, bitter, and blue.

As word continued to spread, I received text messages of love and encouragement and then phone calls of confirmation that they knew in advance that this battle would be won and that cancer had picked the wrong woman to mess with. It gave me hope, and that is what I needed to get through the first few weeks. It seemed surreal, still. Corey was by my side at every appointment. He may not have understood the ins and outs, but he was, for sure, present and available to me for support, encouragement, and just to hold me up when I was too weak.

My mom also played a critical role. I knew she was shaken. I knew this took the wind out of her, so when she was present, I tried to put on a face that I had this and we would be absolutely fine—but Mom always knows. No matter how much I smiled, joked, or attempted to shrug off my feelings, I could look in her eyes and tell that she would be strong for me whenever I needed her to be and that she would be in a fight with me. So much so that she was the first to say, "When you start losing your hair, I'm cutting mine too!"

When I first heard her say it, I thought, *Why would you do something like that? It's totally unnecessary.* But as I got further along in the journey, I learned that many family members and friends did that as a symbolic gesture of love and support of the survivor in their lives. She eventually did cut her hair, and when she did, my heart melted. I felt blessed to not only have my mom present but also to have her completely in my corner, no matter what was required. A mother's love, right?

My mom and I had a rocky relationship during my teen years, especially after my father passed. I loved her, but I didn't like her parenting style when it came to me. In my eyes, she was extremely easygoing on my brother, and he had very few consequences, but for me, she was overly stern and plain-old mean. Well, that's what I used to think. As I matured and life got the best of me, we had a conversation. She told me once, "I push you because I see something in you. You're different, and you're special. You will be better." At the moment, that meant the world to me because I often doubted that she actually believed any of that to be true about me. Over my years on this earth, we've fallen out and haven't seen eye to eye. But to look at us now, it's so different. She shows her love in so many ways. She is always available to me and gets upset if I miss a day of not calling to check on her. She is often at our home to love on the kids and make my favorite meals or desserts. She often takes the kids to give Corey and me a break. And sometimes, we just sit in silence and watch TV together. All things I never thought would happen a few years back.

Cancer seemed to bring us even closer. I realized that no matter how old I got, I always need my mother's love, and I'm blessed that she is still here with me to provide that love. During treatment, she was in the cancer center with me; she asked doctors questions; she made sure that she was not only present but actively engaged in understanding what I needed. She was and still is an amazingly strong woman that would absolutely do anything for me.

I am the youngest of ten siblings. The majority of them are my father's children; in other words, seven of us share a father, and two of us share a mother. Nonetheless, we are siblings, and all of them played a role in my journey. One of my brothers and his wife faithfully came to our house once a week to prepare a meal for us. He pushed me to get off the couch and walk around. Although at the time I hated him for it because I felt like he didn't understand, I understood that his heart was in the place of "I'm not letting you just give up!" My sister-in-law did everything from washing dishes to cleaning bathrooms. It was super-uncomfortable for me, but I deeply appreciated everything they were doing for my family.

My other brothers and sisters went through a period of what I can only describe as denial. It was unreal to them that this was true. In fact, one of my brothers, Tyrone, told me I was telling a lie when I gave him the news. Our family has a traumatic and unfortunate bad history of health issues. Everything from heart disease and high blood pressure to obesity and cancer. All of my siblings supported me in different ways, and I believe it had much to do with how we were raised.

By the time I'd come along, I was ten years behind the last sibling, my dad had shifted and was much more affectionate with me. My father had not been the hug, kiss, soft touches, and conversationalist type. He was an enforcer that made you "lie in the bed you made for yourself." So, that was their approach. They engaged, asked questions, or showed support as I included them or reached out to them to update them on the progress of things. There was a point where this made me bitter and upset. It went back to those expectations I placed on them. In my mind, they should have just stepped up, helped with the kids, provided meals, whatever we needed, but that wasn't the case, and today, I understand and accept that fact.

Even with that being said, I knew I had to grow up and accept the roles I put them in. They didn't necessarily "owe it to me" to be present, and everyone deals with things differently. As my father was not affectionate, neither were they. They didn't mean any harm, and I learned to include them and tell them what I wanted and needed from them. We grew as siblings, and I believed we loved each other a little more deeply too.

Then there is my own personal sister circle. I have a group of seven women that I can call on for just about anything. They were my prayer warriors, encouragers, doctor visit note takers, chemo partners, and so much more.

I recall one day when I was home alone. Corey was at work, the girls at daycare, and Corey Jr. at school. I was struggling. I was angry every time I looked in the mirror, every time I had to dash to the bathroom to vomit, and every time I stepped on the scale to see I'd be down another two to three pounds. I was angry that I felt like I was dying alone. In my mind, I was losing the fight. I had stopped answering the phone and would not respond to text messages. I put my phone on "Do Not Disturb" and sat on the floor and cried like a baby.

I was hurt and spiraling into depression. And then there was a knock at the door, followed by a constant ringing of the doorbell. Whoever was on the other side of the door was not going away. I opened the door to find my girlfriend, Lashonda, standing there with her precious newest edition, baby Alex. Lashonda has a bright and bubbling personality. There is no way to be around her and not laugh; she's a mood changer! She said, "Hold up, I know you are not dodging my phone calls. You obviously don't know who you messing with…where is your phone? Open these shades, what's wrong with you?"

I laughed, but then I sat back down on the floor and said very honestly, "I'm tired of feeling like this. I'm tired of being sick. I'm tired of feeling useless."

And then she handed me Alex. His little face looked up at mine, and his eyes, so pure and honest, smiled and cooed. Tears fell from my face, but this was exactly what I needed at that very moment, to see a little life and recall the little lives in my own life that still needed me to fight. Lashonda snapped a picture of that moment, and I still have it. It was a shift to fight and a realization that I needed to find a way to get out of my head when I'm alone. My friends and family helped me do that.

I made a point after that to answer my phone when I didn't feel like talking, to begin to take walks to allow the sun to shine down on my bald head, to take time to feel the breeze, and to write down the emotions that I held inside.

During chemo, I had to learn to accept the help that was being given. Many of my girlfriends coordinated care, meaning they would determine the best shift to come sit with me while Corey and my mom worked. They often would bring their laptops and join me in my bed. Zundra faithfully made sure I got sunlight by raising the blinds. Brandi ensured I had ginger drops for my nausea and a few aroma-therapy items to choose from. Tracee ensured that I had peace and quiet. Angela made sure I had food. Nikki came to treatment and did drop-ins to make sure I did what Corey told me to do. Tanesha kept me laughing, and Kanisha kept me inspired and always looking forward. Letitia took time out of her day to drive me to doctor appointments and sit with me as long as I wanted her to be there. One word, grateful!

The girlfriend code was in effect, and there was nothing I could do about it, as if I wanted to. These women, in addition to many others, cared for me and carried me in their thoughts and prayers. I am so blessed to know and love these women and to have them love me back.

The last round of chemo treatment, number sixteen, as a matter of fact, I invited a host of family and friends to celebrate the triumph of conquering the first leg of the cancer journey. Corey and I arrived at the chemo center first as I would see my oncologist on this day, and then I would receive treatment. It was August 6, 2019, at about 9:30 a.m. My name was called as usual, and Corey and I walked back to see the doctor to assess my progress and plan for what was coming next, which would be a bilateral mastectomy with the removal of lymph nodes and insertion of expanders.

I took a picture with Dr. Salem and then headed over to the infusion center. As I got hooked up, my family and friends began arriving. It was definitely a moment. I was thankful that they had taken time from their normal Tuesday activities to be present with me and also thankful that the nursing team was being completely flexible as my "team" continued to arrive.

At the conclusion of treatment, my favorite nurse began unhooking me. My eyes shut close, and I began to silently pray. I had Koryn Hawthorn "Won't He Do It" playing on my cell phone. Tears began to fall. In what seemed like the same instance, the nurse began handing out bells to all of the friends and family that decided to take one. I had one of my cousins video calling another cousin so that she would be able to participate in the event. Once I was patched up I made a dart for the wall to ring the bell, I actually rang the bell so hard that I thought it was going to come off the wall! As I turned back around, I fell into Corey's arms, letting out a bellow from deep in my belly. I turned from him and grabbed my mom. From there, all I saw were pleasant faces, most wiping tears, and all cheering and giving praise to God that *we* had made it through.

From that day to this one, I still have my village. It's actually grown. Through the pain, I pushed to love others, and in return, I am loved and supported twice as much. I've had many low moments during the journey, which is expected, but I've also experienced love, laughter, and life in a new and different way. I once heard a quote from Oprah that said, "Lots of people want to ride with you in the limo, but what you want is someone who will take the bus with you when the limo breaks down." Cancer was the limo that broke me down, and I found out what type of friends I was working with!

There are many of us, though, that do not have this same type of testimony. I've heard of several women walking this road alone because they are not fortunate to have support, or they have chosen not to burden others with the misfortune that has come upon their lives. And to those women, I want you to know you are never alone. We choose to isolate ourselves because we had been conditioned for so long to be strong and carry the burdens that happened within our lives. This could not be further from the truth. This disease has run so rapidly that your sister survivors need to hear from you. They need your story as much as you need to be surrounded with people that can hear you and understand the cross you bear.

I encourage you to use your doctors and nurses to help provide you with support group options, and if that isn't your thing (it sure wasn't mine), use social media to connect with others. Sometimes just being a part of a chat where someone is experiencing what I'm experiencing helps to push a little harder and carry on just a little while longer. We are sisters, not bound by blood but of love and testimony. You will live to fight another day. I am here for you whenever you need me to be. You are *not* alone, no matter if you were diagnosed yesterday or twenty-five years ago. You matter to me and all of your survivor sisters. I urge you not to go through this alone. I urge you to take action to build support where you need it.

It isn't always necessary to tell your story. You don't have to share anything, but at some point, everyone needs someone. We were never built to live this life alone, cancer or not!

CaringBridge Journal Entry: Look How Far We Have Come!
Journal entry by Anastasia Stevenson—July 16, 2019

Good morning, Family!
I hope this note finds you happy, healthy and whole! ***long post alert***
I haven't done an update since before the 4th of July which is almost two weeks ago! Crazy! What's more crazy is that I've been on this journey since the mid-February. Let me say it again, we're in mid-July! So here are the updates!

Family: Everyone is doing well. We're preparing for the twins' fourth birthday party this Saturday. On Tuesday, July 23rd, they will be four and this will be a magical birthday… literally…unicorn appearance and everything (yes, I said unicorn)! The realization that I could have died after giving birth to the twins is real to me. Although this is becoming a more & more common story, the fact of the matter is internal bleeding post C-section happened to me. I almost lost my life (once more) which then meant that God isn't through with me! I brought home two little girls, that I thought I wasn't fit to begin to raise, six pounds, ten ounces and five pounds, nine ounces. They were healthy and still are! They are thriving and loving life. They are sassy and filled with love. They are amazing little people that make me laugh, cry and see how beautiful life is…how amazing life is! CJ is the best big brother ever. He recently lived his best life, traveling to Destin, FL with his Granny, uncle Jerry and aunt Lucy. They attended my cousin's wedding and also got in some good beach time and site seeing. What made my heart melt that even in separation and knowing that one of his sisters is a troublemaker (I'll let you guess which), he brought them home a little surprise. He thought of them, he's a great young man! I'm thankful for my mom taking care of him and providing him a great time! I'm blessed. Corey Sr. is still amazing. I can't say enough about how awesome he is and he has been and continues to be. Marriage is hard but with the partner that is willing to fight with you and *for* you...amazing. It feels good to be loved by him and even better to love him and let him know he is loved by me! That's important!

How I'm doing: *Chilllllll*. Let me tell you! God is amazing! I have energy, I have a life, I have love and I have *you!* Each of you that provide encouragement, support and love—even when I'm not thinking or feeling I need it. I was blessed several times over the past two weeks but I have to call out one thing. One of my good friends held a birthday event. *Her* birthday event, where she dedicated time to love on me and in the name of breast cancer education and support. She introduced me to the founder and CEO of The Pink Angels Foundation, Chantelle Nicholson-Clark, who is a nine-year breast cancer survivor. During my friend's event, she asked my permission to share my story... and in the room where *several* survivors that looked like me, one of them shared one of my doctors. I was presented with a love offering, several contacts, an inner circle and *lots of love and prayer y'all!* In addition, for the first time since January, *I worked out!* I'm not talking about stretching and meditation. I'm talking full out Zumba (led by Tracee—who is an amazing teacher), Twerk fitness, boot camp *and* yoga! I didn't do it all but I did *well!* I hung in and felt amazing! So to you Tracee and Chantelle (Pink Angels Foundation), *thank you!* You are absolutely amazing and Happy Birthday, Tracee! Thank you for including me and The Pink Angels Foundation in your amazing life celebration!

What's next? The time we have been waiting on is upon us. After today's chemo treatment, I will have *three* (or less) cycles left. This Friday, I'm scheduled for a rescan of my left breast to assess the three tumors and provide those images to Dr. Vaughan (breast surgeon). Following that I will meet with Dr. Vaughan on Thursday, July 25th, to discuss the plan for the surgery and get it scheduled. As a recap, I'm electing a double mastectomy with full removal of my areola and reconstruction. This will require about two surgeries to complete. I'll also need to complete radiation. After doing the research, this will lower the possibility of recurrence… but that's not the only thing…there's a lesson!

What I'm learning: In that January fast done with my church this year, I asked God to use me and as I'm going through this process, I've had visions and thoughts—unsure of if they are mine or if this is God speaking to me. But I kept saying "But God, I don't have what it takes, I'm scared, I'm fearful, I don't even know if I belong in some of the situations I'm in." I don't know if I deserve to talk to the people that I have met and are now in "my network" or if I'm experiencing the "Impostor Syndrome." I don't know if my voice will work or if this will work out...what about the money, Jesus...how will I do this? And in that session on Saturday with Tracee and Chantelle, Chantelle spoke an awaited word. She said, "Don't pay attention to what's in the bag, God said that when you are faithful over little. He will make you Ruler over much." *Wow, wow, wow!* When I awoke this morning (2:00 a.m.) with no ability to continue sleeping, I ran across a sermon by Sarah Jakes Coleman about being "Empty Handed," I feel like I'm getting my answer...the sermon when something like: there is power in my *empty hands*, and God will restore what the enemy tried to steal, that God is not finished with us yet and that the *power* that is in our hands is more than enough. How *great* is our God. We have room to move as the Lord says so. I can tell you that I'm different. I began to say in this last two weeks, planting a seed, that "Who needs a cure when you have the *healer*!" And beyond that, God—move my feet, I surrender all! I give it all away!

Here, friends, is my transparency. I experienced such a feeling of depression on July 3rd and 4th. I was down; I shed tears and hid them from my husband, close friends, and my family. I suffered in silence, *but* when God moves, *he* moves. He told me to use my hands (before I even heard this sermon). And in that, I re-finished the furniture in the girls' room and changed it completely! I had never done anything like this before… I'm talking sanding, mudding, repairing and painting, two and a half days of *work*. But the end result! My God, the power was in my hands, and I had no idea what I was capable of.

During that work, I prayed, I spoke to God in my words in my plain words, "Father to daughter talk." No ritual, repeated words, or alter needed. I sat at his feet, moving the paintbrush and fellowshipped with my Father, and I believe he heard me. I repented, declared his promises, and made my heart desires known, and day by day, more and more, I hear him…and even when I'm unsure that it is Him, *I move, I listen, I obey.* I'm grateful.

As always, thank you for sticking with me. Thank you for your prayers and keep them coming. I love you. If there is anything I can do, let me know! I'm praying for you. In closing, a few great scriptures:

God is our refuge and strength, an ever-present help in trouble. Therefore we will not fear, though the earth give way and the mountains fall into the heart of the sea, though its waters roar and foam and the mountains quake with their surging. (Psalm 46:1–3 NLT)

The Lord is my strength and my song; he has given me victory. This is my God, and I will praise him—my father's God, and I will exalt him! (Exodus 15:2 NLT)

Those who seek the Lord lack no good thing. (Psalm 34:10 NLT)

You are my hiding place; you will protect me from trouble and surround me with songs of deliverance. (Psalm 32:7–8 NLT)

I tell you the truth, you can say to this mountain, 'May you be lifted up and thrown into the sea,' and it will happen. But you must really believe it will happen and have no doubt in your heart. (Mark 11:23 NLT)

Amen, and it is so! You shall have whatever you say!

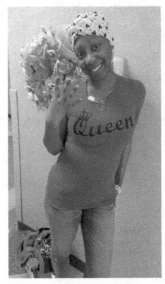

Anastasia at the Cancer Treatment Center on July 9th with four more chemo cycles to go!

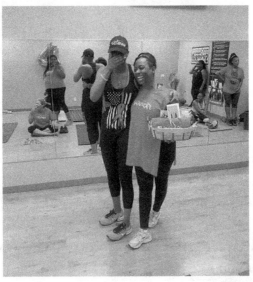

An unexpected surprise & real tears @ Tracee's 40th Celebration Event w/ Founder & CEO The Pink Angels Foundation Chantelle Nicholson-Clark

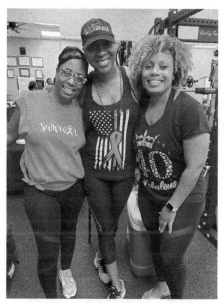

After a full workout... Chantelle, me and
Tracee!!! Love you both, dearly

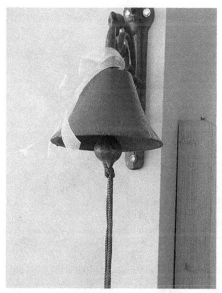

Completion bell in the chemo center...here's
the proof I left it in tact on the wall!

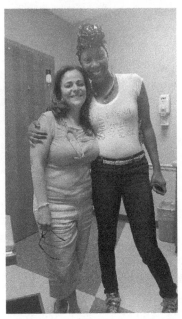

Anastasia and Dr. Salem – Medical Oncologist

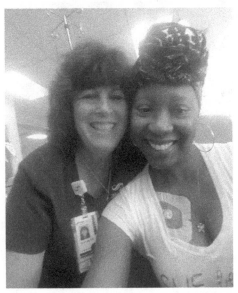

Anastasia and Nurse Jeannie, my favorite chemo nurse!

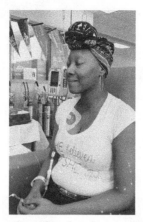

Anastasia in prayer as the takes her last round of chemo, 8/6/20.

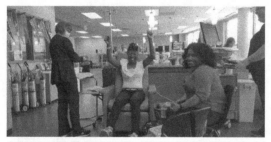

Anastasia & Brandi in celebration!

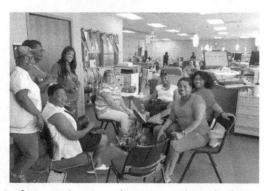

From Left to Right: Standing, Tanesha Gleghorn, Nikki
Brooks, Kanisha Anthony. Sitting Eloise (mom), Barb Koerber,
Anastasia, Brandi Henry & Zundra Bryant. Celebrations at
the last day of Chemo! Not pictured: Tracee Green, Letitia
Avery, Jerry McClendon, Lucy McClendon, Chazsaty Harmon,
Tacarra Thomas, Lashonda Lockhart and Lavell Dean.

Chapter 7

Love and Marriage

"Haven't you read," he replied "that at the begin-
ning, the Creator made them male and female
and said, 'For this reason, a man will leave his
father and mother and be united with his wife,
and the two will become one flesh?' So they are
no longer two but one flesh. Therefore what God
has joined together, let no man separate."
—Matthew 19:4–6 (NLT)

Marriage. I think that one word can be a beginning, middle, and end of this chapter! The truth of the matter is that marriage is work, no matter what winds of life blow. Marriage is also one of the biggest blessings that one might receive. If chosen correctly, you have a built-in friend, partner, strategic advisor, comedian, lover, and caretaker. There are some of us that don't require the certificate, fancy ceremony, and pomp and circumstance, and that's fine; nonetheless, a partner in crime is always a great thing to have.

We go through the courtship, dating all to discover this person just might be what we need to continue to grow. I thought, *I surely could build something with this guy.*

Corey and I met on Myspace.com. For those of you too young or maybe beyond the age of Myspace, it was a more personal version of Facebook. You created your own pages, complete with background graphics, added tons of pictures, and followed friends and met new ones. In our case, Corey "DM'd" (direct messaged) me. He sent a note to my personal inbox, asking if I knew of any hot spots, clubs, or where the parties were as he was new to the Saint Louis area and he wanted to get familiar with what was hot.

My response was, "Nope, I don't go out. I'm not that chic."

He was persistent and somehow was successful in continuing our conversations at first through direct messages only, and then eventually, he sent me his phone number. It was then that I could actually confirm that he was not a native St. Louisian as his area code was 504. That's right, good ol' New Orleans. I hesitated for a couple of days to call Corey, but then I finally did. Right off the cuff, his accent drew me in. It was a typical made-for-TV type situation where we held all of these late-night conversations and chatted about nothing really.

Eventually, we made plans to meet face-to-face, and should our meeting go well, we'd go on a date. For me, my safety was important, so I had Corey meet me in front of my mom's home. He said he'd swing by after he left work on Friday evening. In my mind, here was another chance for me to validate his Myspace profile; namely, do you own a vehicle! I was done at this point with dating guys who did not or could not at least meet me where I was in life. I was far from perfect but trying! I had a full-time job, in school, taking a full-time course load to obtain my bachelor's degree and also taking care of my Godson—full-time!

That Friday evening, Corey called to let me know he was in the area and would be pulling up to the house shortly. As I walked outside, I saw a gold Toyota Tundra approaching the house with a dark-skinned male driving in military uniform. I think the answer in my head was a resounding *Yes!* Nonetheless, this young man got out of the truck, approached the house, and asked if I was Anastasia, to which I replied, "I am" and extended my hand for a handshake.

Corey then took a second to look me up and down and, in verbatim, said, "Oh no, you don't look like your pictures at all. You have acne marks on your face, and what type of skirt is that? No thanks, I'm good." And he proceeded to turn and walk away!

Yes, my chin was on the ground, my eyes had begun to roll, and no words could escape my mouth fast enough, but just as they started to form, he turned back around with a childlike grin, laughing hysterically, saying, "No, no, no, I'm just kidding! I'm Corey."

My face was still expressing the shock and awe from the two seconds prior, but I extended my hand to his to shake his hand. "It's nice to meet you…I think," I responded.

He was still laughing and swore he was just kidding. We make small talk, but my guard was completely up. At the end of the exchange, he said, "I'm going to go home, shower, change, and then I'll be back to pick you up for our date." I didn't believe a word that came out of his mouth, but I told him okay and that I'd see him in about an hour.

Still not believing he was going to show up, I got in and got dressed. No matter if he'd show or not, I would leave the house to go somewhere even if I only went for a drive or to visit family.

He came back, and I told him I'd drive. I didn't trust him, and besides, he didn't know the city that well anyway. We went on to have a great first date—dinner at TGI Fridays, bowling, and then a long walk and talk at Forest Park, near the beautiful fountain pond. We were there for no less than three hours. In fact, the park had closed, unbeknownst to us. When we walked back to the car, there was a ticket on my windshield. Corey grabbed the ticket and told me not to worry about it; he'd take care of it. Yep, that sealed the deal. It wasn't a grand gesture, but by this time, Corey had given me laughter, conversation, interest, and protection.

I drove us back to my mom's house, where he got in his truck and went home. Yes, there was a short peck of a good-night kiss. I'm not sure how far Corey had gotten before my phone rang again. He called to say he had a good time and that he hoped to do it again soon. To which we absolutely did.

Now, I'll spare all of the details, but Corey and I dated for a sum of three years and, in the third year, got married: July 31, 2009. Later in our "dateship," we had issues of fidelity, which spilled into our marriage. Not the infidelity but the lack of trust. I'd begun to guard my heart from him, believing that he couldn't tell as I would still be performing all of my "wifely duties." During the course of our relationship, the military played a big role. I learned during dating that Corey would be spending some weekends, some weeks, possibly even months with his army sisters and brothers. I learned quickly what it meant to be in a relationship with someone that had goals of making the military a career. I packed bags, practiced the "Soldiers Creed," and helped him prepare for promotion boards. Corey would say that it was me that pushed him to do better and to want better for himself, that I made him want to provide for a family and be more for himself and potentially the family that we would one day start. I say it was within him and I just pushed it closer to the surface.

Marriage was hard, especially when you involved family in the fight. It causes rifts, discomfort, and destroys peace.

Several times throughout our marriage, we sought counseling, mentor couples, and worked on ourselves individually. Some things worked better than others, and then something would happen that would set us back. One of those things happened to be a military deployment when our firstborn son was just one year old. There is no handbook for how to work through this—the preparation for the departure, the departure, the time during the deployment, and then the readjustment upon returning home. It was God and God alone that sustained us.

We fought via Skype. I was resentful and even angry that I was home, taking care of our child, back in school for a master's degree, trying to remain married, and yet, feeling very single. We also still had major trust issues, and every time Corey mentioned the name of one particular woman, I cringed. The relationship they'd developed during the deployment made me feel insecure. I think that was because I was fighting to give him what I thought he needed, and he was fighting to try to get me to understand what he actually did need. Listening and communication—powerful lessons to learn in the pursuit of love and happiness.

Fast forward four years, we were now parents of three little ones. The twins were added to our crew on July 23, 2015. During their birth, done via C-section, we had a bit of an issue. About twelve hours after birth, I began to pass out. It was determined that I had internal bleeding, and I needed to be rushed back into surgery. Thank God, my husband was there. He told me he sent the twins to the nursery; his focus was me. He needed his wife to live, and he needed to be completely present. Corey made all the decisions, made the phone calls, and never left my side.

As I slipped in and out of consciousness, I remember seeing his face, I remember him holding my hand and assuring me I'd be okay. I believed him; his eyes always told me the truth. As I went into surgery, I recall telling the anesthesiologist that I needed to live. I had to be there for my babies, and his response was, "You absolutely will! Go ahead and start counting back from ten for me."

I can't tell you what Corey felt or even what his demeanor was, but I know his heart was beating for me. Once surgery was complete, and they began to roll me back up to my room, he grabbed the bed, followed by my mom and one of my brothers. I saw the pain, fear, and panic in all their faces, but God!

I think it was that moment that I knew a major shift had to happen between Corey and me. We needed to work our marriage out, not for our kids but ourselves. We owed it to us to be happy, to be loved, and to be filled by the person we had chosen to take those vows with. We both took them seriously and made the commitment to ourselves and each other that divorce was not an option. I heard somewhere that Will and Jada Pinkett-

Smith also made that commitment to each other, so we were in pretty good company.

Over the course of the four years that followed the twins' entrance to the world, we got better, then fell apart, got better, then fell apart until we were both sick and tired of the cycle. Enter prayer and fasting! December 2018, while at church, the pastor asked the question, "What will you believe God for in 2019?" I sowed a seed of faith and said that this upcoming fast, I would be deliberate and intentional about my marriage. I would surrender what the Word said, and we would get our marriage on the right track—loving, honoring, obeying—everything those marital vows told us we should be. It was also around this time that Corey found out he'd be starting a new role with the government and moving into a reservist role with the army. We were excited about his new start. Additionally, we had also agreed I could begin working on my doctorate degree. Lots of change at one time.

Once the fast began, I was praying and felt nudged to get Corey in on the fast as well. Some days were better than others. I was committed wholeheartedly, but Corey was lukewarm for the process. We journaled together and shared our thoughts, and we prayed together as well. At the end of the fast, I could see small changes, but I was definitely wanting so much more. Then February came. I found the lump, and life was instantly different. Corey was just as solid as he was the night of the internal bleeding, but this time, even more stoic, firm, and completely bought in. No matter what I felt, how many tears I cried, he was there, reassuring, confident, and God was on our side.

We had serious conversations that some things needed to come off of my plate. The battle that was ahead would not allow me to keep moving at the same pace I had been moving. I am a hands-on mom that had the kids in activities. We were solid in church, and both of us were working hard at work in addition to the new doctoral courses I began taking. We agreed that school would be put on hold, and the kids' activities would decrease. The beauty is that they would still be able to participate in activities that were offered at school and daycare.

It was through the breast cancer journey that our marriage had evolved into something new and beautiful. We both had the thought, inspiration, and even encouragement that there was so much more to love and marriage, but neither of us could get through, pass, or get over the hang-ups that had happened over the course of our now thirteen-year relationship. Now, those things didn't matter. I needed him, and he needed me. We learned to put all that advice to work when the rubber met the road.

I began to communicate, telling him what I needed; not every time was executed perfectly. He showed up for me in ways that I didn't know that he could. He chose me over everything. I knew he had done this before, but there was a different glow to it. Maybe my eyes had just been opened a little wider.

As treatment began, he worked with his new employer to work from home on Tuesdays and Wednesdays as Tuesday was treatment day and Wednesday happened to be the day that treatment would begin to kick my butt. We called in reinforcements when necessary, days when management needed Corey in the office. The funny thing, though, was that no matter what person was there, I craved for the support, love, and attention from Corey and Corey only. He was the only person who, no matter how sick I was or how grey my skin appeared, didn't panic. He was confident that this moment would pass.

One day, in particular, Corey had been at work. I was having an awful day. Every muscle in my body hurt from vomiting. I couldn't hold any food, crackers, or sip any water—nothing was comfortable, and I was too exhausted to try to get upstairs to bed. My mom was with me, and so was my best friend, Brandi. They did everything they could for me. I mostly slept. But when Corey came through the door, exhausted, I'm sure from his day at work, he darted to me. He got down on his knee and whispered, "I'm going to change my clothes, and I'm coming right back to you. I love you."

I looked at him with tears forming in my eyes and waited. In basketball shorts and a T-shirt, he sat on the floor next to me, and it's like my body instantly became glued to him. I laid my head in his lap and wrapped my arms around his waist, balled up in the fetal position. He grabbed a blanket and tucked it around me, and I fell swiftly into a peaceful sleep. It was as if all I needed was him, his presence, and his warm embrace. When I shifted to get up to run to the bathroom, he was right behind me, rubbing my back and letting me know it was going to pass, it was going to be okay.

This was our constant: His presence of peace. He prayed over me and tucked me in. He laid with me on the floor and picked me up out of the shower once when I almost fainted. He washed me and wiped me. He was truly in the depths of "in sickness and in health." Through every chemo treatment, Corey sat near with his laptop on his lap and sometimes stepped out to take conference calls so as not to disturb the other patients. At every doctor's appointment, he wiped tears and calmed my fears. He held my hand and squeezed it to remind me that he was there and I was not in the fight alone. There were times when I told him, "No, I'm fine, I can do this appointment alone," only to walk out into the waiting room to see him sitting, waiting on me to receive an immediate update.

At each surgery, he was my chauffeur and main caretaker. He distributed my meds and filled ice packs. He had conversations with family and held the house down as best as he could. He woke up in the middle of the night with work the next morning because he sensed I was awake. He calmed my fears and spoke to my anxiety and wiped my tears. We became so ingrained with one another that in times where I was feeling completely weak, at my end, and done with the whole thing, Corey would be my calm. Other times, I was strong so that Corey could let out his feelings. We relied on each other heavily. It was a total God-synced situation. Every time I looked into his eyes, I could feel nothing but thankfulness.

I chuckle looking back at some of the conversations I had with my girlfriends around the dialog of marriage. Of course, they knew that cancer was having a dramatic effect on our relationship, but the underlying question was "Is it impacting '*every*' area of the relationship?" The answer was yes! You see, what she really wanted to ask is, "I know, for a man, sex is much of the relationship, so how are you handling that, my dear?"

Sex is one of the topics that I don't think is ever mentioned or talked about in a positive light within, from my experience, the black community. Girls are told not to engage while males are told to sew your royal oats. Then in the middle, somewhere, girls become promiscuous, and males are just being boys. However, that's a tangent for another book.

Breast cancer, in and of itself, was a complete struggle. When we throw in marriage and "marital acts," there's a whole other level of struggle. Corey didn't add pressure or even make many advances, trying to encourage sex by any means, knowing and seeing what I was going through on a daily basis. The good thing—if there was a good thing—about going through my chemo regimen was that I had one week in between treatments on the first three medications. This one week gave me a break to almost feel like myself, and it would be during that week that Corey and I would have some sort of intimacy. It did not always lead to sex, but when it did, it was great for both of us. For me, it provided reassurance that no matter how much weight I lost, the change in my complexion, or baldness of my head, my husband still wanted and enjoyed all of me.

For Corey, he wanted and needed sex! No more, no less. We had an unspoken understanding, and sometimes I question how he remained attracted to me. All I saw was baldness, my clothes falling off me because of my decreasing weight, my chemo port that stuck out of my chest, and my shifting complexion signifying the changes in my blood cells and the impact of chemo drugs. His response was that he fell in love with me, and no matter my weight or what changes my body undertook, his heart for me remained the same, but what he needed in return was to feel just as loved, just as accepted, and just as appreciated.

So yes, we engaged in sex. There were no special modifications needed. My challenge during engagement was to remain present in the moment and not allow my mind to drift to my circumstances or medical diagnosis. I was still me, and he was still him. It took some practice, and through every phase, this, too, improved. What's more ironic about it all is that now that we're closely approaching the other side of the journey, both of us now want more out of our sex lives, not just because, let's face it, it feels good, but more because the connection and bond formed through sex is intoxicating. It makes us want to be around each other more. We can't pass each other in the hall or walk near each other without some sort to touch of embrace. That connection is rare but also necessary. Love lives there, and where there is love, there is life!

We sit and talk sometimes and discuss the past year and the impact that it's had on our relationship and life in general. We discuss the hard times, but we spend even more time reflecting on the good. It can become so easy to just see the negative in the situation, the road most traveled, but it takes intention to really look at the positive things that were birthed through that difficult road. While chatting one evening, I explained to him that I began looking at him as my hero through this process. I mean, he literally has picked me up off the bathroom floor more times than I care to count. The times that he sat with me on the floor, because it was the most comfortable place for me, were amazing, romantic, and so sweet. For him, I later found out it was convenient. He wouldn't have to continue going back and forth, and he could be there if I needed something. It was an opportunity for him to rest, as well.

When we were at the cancer treatment center and doctor's appointments for me, he was my strength. He kept me calm and supported me. For him, in those times, I made him feel like he could handle it. He told me he never knew where he got the energy to keep going. He explained it was a God thing. He felt like if he could just keep moving, then God would give him the strength and will to keep going and get things done. He also said that he tried to keep up with the house chores because he knew that if the house was sort of clean, I would be a little more at ease. We both had needs that were being met through each other but not the same ideas of how they impacted us. Nonetheless, the love was shown, and it reaped dividends more.

The lessons we learned through the journey have been plentiful. They have allowed us to see each other's point of view and not attempt to make things what the other person believes they should be. We learned the importance of good communication and how imperative complete honesty is within the relationship. We often cue conversations with "can I be honest," which lets other person know that there is a dialog that needs to happen, and we cannot be guarded and needed to lean in with our hearts and not our heads. We've learned each other's value, and that even if the house is clean, it's a miserable place to be when you're not speaking to the other resident! Our resolves happen faster, and we are a partnership. I've learned to help in all areas of the house, including cutting the grass. I actually find it to be relaxing and an easy way to get a workout in!

I believe Corey would agree with me when I tell you that breast cancer saved our marriage. Before this happened, we heard each other but didn't listen. We existed together but never engaged well. We had fights and no resolution to arguments! All those muscles were flexed through this evolution of me. So many things I had to deal with internally, including my confidence, expressing love, and leaning into trust—trust in the man that I married.

I had no indication that breast cancer would interrupt our lives and also had no indication that breast cancer would quite possibly save my marriage, but it did. We are better, wiser, and stronger than I imagined could be possible. It's like the twelve-month journey added another five years to our marriage. We're far from perfect and still have issues here and there, but the resolutions are faster, the love is deeper, and the peace is in abundance. I know for sure that I am his, and he is mine.

CaringBridge Journal Entry: New Week New Goals
Journal entry by Anastasia Stevenson—June 19, 2019

Hey, Family!

I pray this update finds you happy, healthy, and whole! It's mid-month...have you done your self-breast exam??? Need to know how? Call ya girl! So, let's get started! I meant to write this update on Saturday night, but here we are on Wednesday!

First off, I'd like to take a moment to shout out my wonderful, supportive, out-standing, amazing husband! Father's Day was good to us! I hope he felt the love from us. As you know Corey has been riding this wave with me. He's been a fantastic cheerleader, coach, encouragement, head shaver, back rubber, chemo partner, tear wiper...well, the list goes on and on. I'm extremely blessed to have his covering—his love, his heart! I'm for-ever grateful to him. I was told in the begin-ning that marriages either grow or fall apart under this type of pressure. In our case, the pressure is producing diamonds! It's amazing, and every day we're able to look at each other and say—yep, we've grown! Growth is imper-ative; going through the suck to see the sun shine again! We're also blessed to have family that prays for us...for that, we thank each of you. Happy Father's Day again, my love!

On the cancer front, we're nine cycles complete and seven to go to complete chemo! We're just over halfway there to complete phase one! The next phase that I've loving named "Get It the Hell *Out* Phase 2" shall kick off in August. I don't have a date for surgery yet but I should have it no later than July 25th! Chemo sessions are getting better. We have found a premed cycle that has been working great. I receive several medicines prior to chemo meds begin to drip and it's been decreasing the sick time dramatically. With continued prayers, I'm hoping I can get my white blood cell count back in the normal range...this one is a major hurdle, but I'm confident we'll get there.

This week's pictures are Corey and I post-treatment yesterday and one pic during treatment. I have a thousand blankets because I have ice on my hands and feet. The chemo drug that I am on tends to cause neuropathy (numbing/tingling of the fingers and toes). It can be temporary or permanent. By God's grace, it's been minimal and the ice has been helping...along with continuing to do normal activity, namely still braiding the girls' hair every week.

I leave you with this verse to run the race that has been set before you...heads up!

Therefore, since we are surrounded by such a huge crowd of witnesses to the life of faith, let us strip off every weight that slows us down, especially the sin that so easily trips us up. And let us run with endurance the race God has set before us. We do this by keeping our eyes on Jesus, the champion who initiates and perfects our faith. Because of the joy awaiting him, he endured the cross, disregarding its shame. Now, he is seated in the place of honor beside God's throne. (Hebrews 12:1–2 NIV)

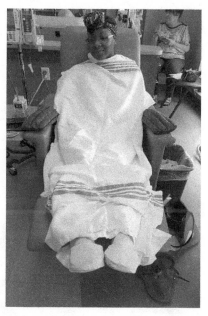

Chemo Treatment #9! Ice packs and blankets!

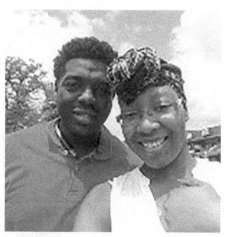

Corey and Anastasia post treatment. Happy Father's Day, my Love!

Chapter 8

There Is Still Life to Live

Surely goodness and mercy will follow
me all the days of my life.
—Psalms 23:6 (NLT)

One thing that I know for sure is that life is promised to no one. As the days continue, we hear about babies leaving the earth as much as we hear that people of older age are. It's in those times where I take a moment to begin to count my blessings to see, understand, and lean into the fact that I am here and present on purpose. We've all endured countless issues, problems, and situations where we may reflect and wonder how we made it out. Breast cancer was that for me.

As time continues to move forward, I often take deep breaths to feel my chest rise and fall; life and life abundantly is what the Word spoke to me. Specifically, the Word says, "The thief cometh not, but that he may steal, and kill, and destroy: I came that they may have life, and may have it *abundantly*" (John 10:10 AMP; emphasis mine). There is a point in life where we make a decision to live the life we have been given rather than to just exist within the world that we've been born into.

I'm confident that there is so much more to life than getting into some mundane routine. There is more to your calling and purpose. You are called to grow beyond the normal by serving and being of service to others. I'm not saying that you need to change careers, change spouses, or anything of the sort, but rather tap into your natural gifts, maybe coaching, mentoring, rocking babies at a local hospital, or baking goodies for local senior centers. The point is there is something great within you, and it's your job to uncover, explore, and evolve.

I was not at all certain that I would make it through the battle. I wasn't sure that I would be present for my kids, so I gave them big parties for their birthdays and showered them with love and affection in case I would not be around any longer. What type of love was that? It was selfish. It was more for me than it was for them. I learned that this is the type of love that they should receive every day, not just in case something happens that is major. There is no love like that of a parent to their children, and in that, you should pray, teach, and love more than anything else. It is a decision to change behavior, modify approach, and lean into a different level of understanding.

I'd canceled myself and took myself out of the game without completely understanding what I was dealing with, the implications, or the possibilities. Looking back, I was driving the car blindfolded, hoping that someone would guide me through it, blocking the vision, the possibilities, initially, and then finally growing into "*I am more.*" I wrote out affirmations, journaled, got involved in and out of the house, stopped my daily routine, and engaged in the dialog instead of just listening. I stopped being passive and started playing the lead role in determining how this thing was going to go. Yes, there are times when I got discouraged, but I didn't stay there.

That's the challenge, to know that you have every right to feel your feelings, but *you cannot stay there!* When I changed, my situation had to change. I smiled during my chemo treatments, eventually, and chatted with the other people that were on a journey of their own. I let them in, and they let me in. I prayed and allowed the Holy Spirit to speak to my heart when I could not.

Day-to-day can be difficult. I've had the final reconstruction surgery, and one might say that like Humpty Dumpty, I've been put back together again. But there are times when I look in the mirror and I don't like what I see. I still deal with the acceptance of my scars where my nipples should be. I fight with the thought that if I wanted to have more kids, my reproduction system won't work, and if it did, I wouldn't be able to breastfeed my babies, should they survive the pregnancy. I also learned that to be the most aggressive in attempting to prevent the return of cancer, it would be best to have a complete hysterectomy, completely removing the chance of having another pregnancy, if we wanted one. I walked through the emotional turmoil of reflecting on difficult times when I was too weak to walk, cook dinner, or even play with my kids. I'm not sure it ever goes away.

While sitting with my sister survivors during group, we talked about those feelings with open and honest dialog. We discussed the potential of the cancer returning, and for some of them, it never left. It's a tough road to walk, but it's not without victory—the victory in our smiles, our continued will to fight, and the desire to turn the pain into purpose. It is in the lives we live every day and each time I walk in my office or mentor a young lady. My calling now has more meaning. It has more power, and it has a renewed sense of urgency.

It's safe to say you don't think the same or process feelings the same. You don't argue the same or even get upset at the same things. You tend to look over the small stuff and even not pay attention to certain things anymore. You grow past pettiness and shift into power and persistence, the persistence that was there all along but now has a new sense of determination. Defeat wasn't an option then, and now it's even more essential to move into purpose, into life, and into passionate responsibility.

For me, the calling in life became a little louder. Not everyone will have that same experience. Life is enough. Being with family and friends one more day is enough. In my case, and in the case of a few other women I have had the pleasure of knowing, this disease became a vehicle of motivation that will push us to desire more for the rest of our lives. The basics aren't good enough. We love harder, breathe deeper, talk with passion, and inspire change. We listen a little more intently and give more freely. We learned there is so much more to do and be and give. There is more love to share and smiles to bring. There is more beyond the shadow of a doubt. There is more!

CaringBridge Journal Entry: Surgery is complete
Journal entry by Anastasia Stevenson—January 16, 2020

Hi, Family!
The last surgery is complete! Yesterday, we completed reconstruction and removed

my chemo port. The surgery went extremely well. Unfortunately, due to how bad the radiation burn was on the left side, the doctor had to make a new incision underneath the breast. He was able to use the same on the left.

Today, I'm really sore, so I'm icing a lot. I did go to my follow-up appointment this morning, and we were happy with the results. I still have a bunch of healing to do, but I'm moving in the right direction.

Thank you for your prayers! Love you all!

Anastasia

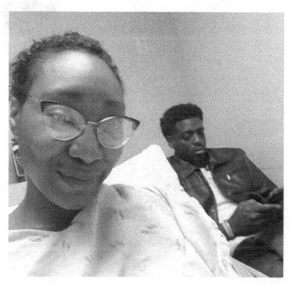

Anastasia & Corey waiting on surgery to begin to replace expanders with implants!

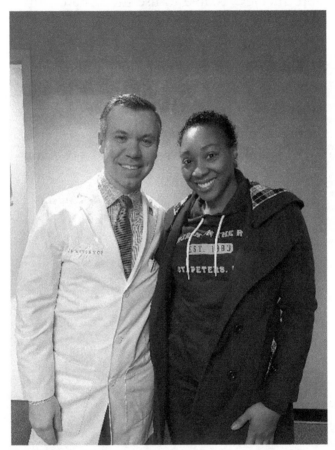

Anastasia & Dr. Mills post reconstruction surgery visit, All good!

Chapter 9

Closing Thoughts

Be confident of this, that He that began a
good work in you will carry it on to com-
pletion until the day of Jesus Christ.
                            —Philippians 1:6 (NLT)

The definition of *evolution*, according to Webster's
Dictionary, is 1. the process by which different kinds of
living organisms are thought to have developed and diversified
from earlier forms during the history of the earth; 2. the gradual
development of something, especially from a simple to a more
complex form.

It's hard work making a conscious choice to dig deep, take
risks, move beyond comfort zones, and do the hard things that
you maybe didn't believe were possible. Something as simple as
speaking up in a meeting, letting your voice be heard could be

the start of something greater. Let me reiterate that this is not a call to go beyond borders and feed everyone on the planet, but if you have an idea, do it! The only thing stopping you is you. You were created as a masterpiece in God's eyes, and there is nothing and no one that is able to change that. The Word says, "So God created mankind in his own image, in the image of God he created them; male and female he created them" (Genesis 1:27 NLT).

So then the question becomes, how do you view God, and how do you interact with him? He is as much of the evolution as you allow him to be. So, I ask, who is God in your life? Is he a far-off bigger-than-life person that watches over you? Or is he with you every step of the way, living within you, breathing through you, and whispering to you all of the answers to the questions that you have to ask him? Only you can make that decision, and based on that decision, you will have that much success with your evolution.

It may seem that the closer you get to the end or the closer you get toward the victory, the less supported you feel. You may begin to feel alone. It's important to acknowledge the emotional aspect of things and pinpoint what brings you to the place of loneliness. For me, it was being alone at appointments and no longer having my family and close friends accompanying me to ensure that I'm on the right path to being healed and healthy.

I recall on one particular day, I had three appointments—physical therapy, plastic surgeon, and radiation. I learned that the radiation appointment would be canceled because, at the time, I still had my drain in. The radiation team informed me that they could not begin working with me until all of the wounds had begun the healing process in the area where the radiation would take place, which in hindsight makes perfect sense. My plastic surgeon told me this would likely be the case, that I would need to reschedule radiation until my sizing was confirmed complete.

Anyway, that morning, Corey and I missed each other and had a spat (in the words of my great-grandmother who taught me that this is the equivalent of a small disagreement). My request to him prior to today was to tell me the night before if our morning routine needed to shift. This day, he woke me up with the change he'd like me to take all the kids into school. No big deal, right? Wrong! Because I felt my request of him to tell me the night before had gone ignored, it frustrated me. Not only did I need to rethink my morning and the timing of things, but I hadn't planned to have an emotional reaction to going to all of my appointments alone. Initially, I was okay because my mom said she'd be going with me, but then she texted me to let me know she would not, when in reality, she asked me if I needed her, and my response was, "No, I'm fine."

So, I had essentially lied to three people—my husband, my mom, and myself. I went about the morning on the newly adjusted schedule and was really quiet. After I dropped off the kids, I had an extra fifteen minutes, so I grabbed a coffee and a bagel. As I got to physical therapy, I paused and sat in silence in the car and opened the Bible app on my phone. Today's verse was Jude 1:20–21 (NLT), "But dear friends, must build each other up in your most holy faith, pray in the power of the Holy Spirit and await the mercy of our Lord Jesus Christ, who will bring you eternal life. In this way, you keep yourselves safe in God's love."

This was my cue. I humbled myself and sent Corey a text to apologize for my overreaction. Not just apologizing but also acknowledging my selfishness and also not letting him in on my feelings and emotions. It was then that I realized we needed each other, but neither of us took the time to say the words that the other one needed to hear. I mentioned that story to highlight that many times, our emotions are lying to us. We make up stories in our head and tell them to ourselves that things are one way when they actually aren't that way. When we feel alone, it's usually because we've isolated ourselves and are not being honest with those that we need to be honest with.

Breast cancer taught me that my family is second only to God. "He must be one who manages his own household well, keeping his children under control with all dignity" (1 Timothy 3:4). There is no work obligation that is able to keep me from being what they need me to be. It taught me that as long as I have God, there is nothing keeping me from anything that I desire—"on asking, and you will receive what you ask for. Keep on seeking, and you will find. Keep on knocking, and the door will be opened to you" (Matthew 7:7)—and that there is nothing that is too hard for me to overcome—"I have told you these things, so that in me you may have peace. In this world, you will have trouble. But take heart! I have overcome the world" (John 16:33).

Every test and trial, every setback or delay, every tear that was cried will never be wasted. Through the process of learning about cancer, now I'm able to educate and advocate for others. Through my pain, I can understand and stand with other women and men that may walk in those shoes. For my children, they will understand what it means and looks like to have compassion, empathy, and love for others. Nothing is wasted. I have gone through an awesome renovation of mind, body, and spirit. Is it perfect? Absolutely not, but I am still evolving. There is more to come, and there will continue to be more as I continue to breathe.

Evolution is not a one stop shop. It's a continual progression of learning, trying, failing, winning, growing, healing, forgiving, releasing, and so much more. Nothing in life stays the same, so why would your every day be the same? Why would you continue to live in the mental space of lack, uncertainty, depression, anxiety, or negativity? You decide. Decide today that you will not only survive, you will thrive! I love the quote by T. E. Lawrence. He says, "All men dream, but not equally. Those who dream by night in the dusty recesses of their minds, wake in the day to find that it was vanity: but the dreamers of the day are dangerous men, for they may act on their dreams with open eyes, to make them possible."

I dare you to dream, go beyond the normal everyday activity, to look inside and discover there is more to you than what the eye can see or even what you feel. You see, feelings are fleeting; they change like the wind!

As I got closer to the end of the rigorous journey, I had my final reconstruction surgery. I opted for implants rather than a flat chest or using silicone inserts and padded bras. I walked into the hospital with confidence. The sun was shining, and my smile could be seen miles away. I was nervous before surgery, and before they wheeled me in, I said a silent prayer that God would make me who he wanted me to be, and I would spend my days serving him and telling my story of how faithful he'd been to me and my family through this process. You see, I was off work for about five months. We never missed a bill. We always had food to eat, and the kids were well taken care of; my employer was understanding, even empathetic to my family and me. No matter what I felt, God took care of us. I met wonderful people, I got out of my comfort zone, I found healing and forgiveness for things that had been done to me in my past, and in some ways, I played a part in bringing my extended family closer together.

I found a village and was able to encourage and inspire other people. I still mentored and engaged with others. I learned more about myself over the course of eleven months, things I never could have imagined. I found strength, tenacity, love, tenderness, and bravery. On this day, I celebrated how far I'd come. As I woke up in recovery, I kept repeating, "We did it, we beat it!" As I went home, I was proud, and it almost felt surreal that we'd made it this far.

In February 2019, January 2020 felt like it was forever away, but I kept going, and I kept growing. I kept pushing and I kept praying, and people kept praying for me. Never underestimate the power of prayer!

In the beginning of the book, I mentioned a couple of things that I had asked God for in the fast of 2019. Turns out all of those prayers were answered, and here are the details:

1. Rebuild my marriage on a solid foundation. The challenge we faced, we faced it together. We went through the fire, held hands, and PUSHed (Prayed Until Something Happened) through to the other side of breast cancer. We had a breakthrough in communication, vulnerability, and our friendship. We pray together, confide in each other, and trust each other like never before. Our hope is renewed in each other and our marriage. As I mentioned, we're not perfect, but we're leaps and bounds from where we were. I don't believe there is anything that can separate us.

God created the bond between us, and we are committed to only growing and nurturing that bond. "For I am persuaded, that neither death, nor life, nor angels, nor principalities, nor powers, nor things present, nor things to come, nor height, nor depth, nor any other creature, shall be able to separate us from the love of God, which is in Christ Jesus our Lord" (Romans 8:38–39).

2. Be the example and help lead my children to Christ. My faith has kept me! It's been the source of strength, love, hope, perseverance, and peace. My children are now part of that experience. We listen to the kids' version of the audio Bible, and they participate in worship and praise. We pray with them every night and most mornings before we separate to go to work and school. They often find Corey and I sitting and either watching or listening to sermons. Sometimes they join us, and other times, Kennedi just smiles at us and tells us, "You guys are so cute" as only a four-year-old can! They often hear me worshipping and giving praise and now know and understand that my tears when praying aren't sad tears, they're happy tears, so they come around me and give me hugs. "Train up a child in the way he should go, And when he is old he will not depart from it" (Proverbs 22:6).

3. My next thing was to reunite my broken family. While we don't talk every day, I can say that my relationships with my family are different. I had to realize that it's not my burden to carry to ensure that everyone in the family gets along. It is my responsibility to do what I can for me. I had to forgive and even ask for forgive-

ness. I humbled myself and did that. I started calling, I started texting and reaching out, and so did they. The change that I wanted to see started with me. It was a sobering feeling to understand, accept, and acknowledge that the issues that I felt we had were just as much my fault as it was theirs. They didn't owe me anything, and I wasn't entitled to anything. If I wanted change, I had work to do, and I did my work (in my best Iyanla Vanzant voice)! "Let love be genuine. Abhor what is evil; hold fast to what is good" (Romans 12:9).

4. Finally, I wanted to have God to heal the hurts of my past. Breast cancer gave me clarity and allowed me the opportunity to get a clearer perspective of what mattered and what did not. It's not that I will forget the things that have happened in my past, but I have been freed and released from the burden that I carried. It was almost like I held on to those things as a badge of survival, but they only weighed me down. Through prayer and the release to God, I don't feel trapped by those things anymore. I understand that I'm only given one shot at life, and I choose how to live that life. God gives me options every day when I wake up. I can choose to be thankful and walk in his grace and mercy, or I can choose to harden my heart and go through life, feeling defeated. My eyes were opened. "Bear with one another and, if one has a complaint against another, forgive each other; as the Lord has forgiven you, so you also must forgive" (Colossians 3:13).

In a sermon given by Bishop T. D. Jakes entitled "I Didn't Know I Was Me," he explains that the emotional roller-coaster ride that we go on is often an indication that you are going through transition. Being unsteady emotionally displays the place you're in is not the place where you are supposed to be. You have to continue through the pressing, beating, and shaking in order to arrive at the person that God intended you to be. As I continue the walk, I reflect and look back on what I've been through. There are times when I feel unsteady, uncertain, and emotionally out of control. Bishop Jakes further explains that our feelings cannot be trusted. They will lie to us and deceive us as they are a conglomerate of our history! They are a response to what has happened in the past, not what will happen in our future. How comforting to know that it's supposed to be that way.

If it were all lined up right, I'd have no purpose of faith, no mission to pursue, and no purpose to walk out. If we were all nice and pretty, tied with a bow, what kind of testimony would I be able to give? What hope would I be able to share? Or how would I be able to be encouraging to anyone else? Our lives are meant to be shared with others. It's meant to be of service and serve others in good times but more in bad or difficult times. The seasons will always change, and some winters will be more harsh than others, but if we hold tight, lean into our faith, and trust God that this will pass, the season will change, and that trial will evolve into a testimony.

Even though the chemo treatments have stopped, I no longer see the radiologist on a daily basis, and my appointments with the oncologist and breast surgeon are now on three-month regimens, I still have struggles. I still long to know what the future holds for me. I know too, though, that it is my responsibility to live, laugh, and love. I know that it is my responsibility to continue to dream, speak, and share my journey. There are days that I feel completely defeated and that I don't belong. I wonder what God has in store for me since he spared my life. I continue to battle with depression and anxious thoughts. *But* I fight. The battle is not over as long as I have breath in my body. I will shout it from the mountaintops that we have new life and life that we shall live abundantly.

We have a duty and obligation to ourselves and no one else to go beyond the norm, to dig deep, to draw from the well that is our Savior and seek him for our "next!" It can absolutely be hard not to stay in a "state of stuck." It can be difficult to move beyond darkness and doubt. In those times, I encourage you to just speak a positive word, write it down, and believe that word. It may be love or joy, peace, or *Jesus!* Speak it over and over until you feel your mood shift. Do the thing that you don't feel like doing. So many days when I didn't feel like writing or feel like I didn't have the words, I didn't feel like it would make a difference, but I pressed on. As I hit one key and word after word started to fill the pages, I felt more encouraged and inspired to speak to you. We are given a choice to fight or not to fight. A choice to stay the same or grow. A choice to continue or to stop. And at the appointed time, the things that you have worked so hard for will begin to manifest themselves.

There is no timing that is more perfect than the timing of God. I didn't choose cancer, it chose me, but I did choose what I would do with it. I would lend my voice to the situation. I would encourage, empower, and give hope. I would shine in times of darkness, and I would get up after every fall.

One of my favorite authors, Brene Brown, said "I'm slowly learning how to straddle the tension that comes with understanding I am tough and tender, brave and afraid, strong and struggling-all of these things, all of the time. I'm working on letting go of having to be one or the other and embracing the wholeness of wholeheartedness" (*Rising Strong*, Brene Brown).

I couldn't say more eloquently that this is part of the evolution. For so many of us, we feel and think we have to be one or the other—only black and white with no shades of gray. I plead with you to shift from that perspective. Being afraid doesn't void your bravery, and being tender doesn't mean you can't be tough. There is room to sway, to move, to grow…to evolve.

> CaringBridge Journal Entry: Today Marks a Year—Reflections
> Journal entry by Anastasia Stevenson—February 6, 2020
>
> Good morning, Family!
> I pray this note finds you happy, healthy, and whole!
> I'm a bit conflicted today. One year ago today, I found a lump in my breast and it shook my world, turned it upside down and yet in the process made my world a little better. Some days I'm completely bitter, angry, and downright depressed. Other days, I'm upbeat, optimistic and empowered…then there are times when I don't know what I'm feeling, I just know I need to get through the day. This week, I will complete two weeks back at work. It has not been easy. I felt as though I needed to come in ready to hit the ground running and take on everything that has been thrown my way. That left me

defeated and broken. The process of pretending that everything is all good, that all is well…yeah that didn't work at all! I came to the realization that I'm still only (at the time) two weeks post-op and have not adjusted to my new normal so to pretend that everything was fine was the biggest lie I could tell myself and anyone around me. I still hurt, I am still processing what I've gone through, and I need help.

I'm grateful for Corey, though. He always has my best interest at heart and forces me to talk when I don't want to. He forces me to get out of the house when I don't feel like it and forces me to accept his love when I feel most unlovable. We watched a sermon two nights ago by Bishop Jakes and then one by Sarah Jakes Coleman. Essentially, the messages were to keep moving and *get up!* I had been going through the motions but not actually seeking the word that I need to give me what I need to be balanced and in alignment with my heavenly Father. Within the two weeks, I'd dropped my self-care routine because I was so tired from work, shifted from the right things to old bad habits. The immediate first thought was *What did you learn from what you've been through?* I needed to reflect on the lessons! There were many but the top three are God, then me then family, boundaries and priorities! It doesn't matter what others think or feel about my life and what their expectations are, I need to move at the pace of me!

I'm seeking counseling (I should have done that a long time ago) because I realize I need some additional tools to help me heal. You can take care of the outside all you want but if the inside is broken, the outside serves no real purpose. I remember that I needed to kill some things inside of me in order to live. That is still the case!

Just as an update, my post-op visits are progressing well. I'm still on weight restrictions on how much I can carry/lift. The wounds are healing well with no signs of infection. My body is still adjusting to the implants. Throughout the day, I have to massage to stop the tingling sensations, which are nerve endings regenerating. I'll have follow-ups with the breast surgeon and oncologist next month. I'm in the final few chapters of the book and plan to submit it to Christian Publishing on Valentine's Day for their review and feedback. I'm nervous and excited! As I already mentioned, I'm back in the office and getting back in the swing of things with some modifications (no logging in late at night—boundaries)!

One last thing, will you say a prayer for my brother, Jerry. He had a minor stroke last night and is in the hospital now. Our family is strong, and so is my faith, but extra prayers would be great! Thank you for being with me on this journey from then to now. For praying for us, giving us your hearts and help, we are grateful. Counting my blessings, not my problems!

Scripture on my heart today is an oldie but a goodie:

[b]eing confident of this, that he who began a good work in you will carry it on to completion until the day of Christ Jesus. (Philippians 1:6)

I love you. Have a great day!

Anastasia!

Helpful Hints

During Chemo

    Gin—Gins hard candy for nausea.

    For medications that increase the likelihood of neurop-
        athy, use ice packs on both hands and feet. *During*
        chemo cycles:

    Sunshine and natural light boost mood and energy.

    If you have bone pain, take one Claritin a day.

    Keep your skin thoroughly moisturized.

    Don't go to the doctor alone, if possible. Support will get
        you through the unexpected emotional highs and lows.

    If you begin to have a metal taste in your mouth, stop
        using regular utensils and use plastic. Do not eat
        anything that comes out of a can.

    When you look good, you feel good. Dress up when you
        don't feel like it, and accessorize with head wraps. I
        used Pinterest and YouTube to learn different ways
        to tie my wraps.

    Stay away from nail salons! It's temporary.

Listen to your body and stay hydrated with plenty of
water. If you are unable to hold water down, call
the treatment center and ask for saline. Hydration
is key!

Always have hard candy on hand. It helps with nausea—
peppermints, gin—gins, etc.

During Radiation

Moisturize *after* treatment and several times during the
day.

For darker skin types, I recommend NERAK lotion, can
be found at https://www.neraknaturalessence.com/.

Lindi Skin Cooler Pads for cooling skin (Amazon).

Wear clothes that you don't mind getting stained with
lotions and oils.

Wash with non-harsh soaps I used Shea Moisture Black
Castor soap.

Surgery—Bilateral Mastectomy and Reconstruction

Rent a lift chair! There are also nonprofits that pro-
vide them. Check your local breast cancer support
groups.

Take it easy!

Zip front sports bras are highly recommended.

Request physical therapy with a breast cancer specialist
within the network.

Water, water, water.

My Playlist—"Time to Fight"

"Surrounded (Fight my Battles)"—Michael W. Smith

"Let the Church Say Amen"—Andre Crouch

"I'll Trust You, Lord"—Donnie McClurkin

"I Call You Faithful"—Donnie McClurkin

"The Battle Is the Lord's"—Yolanda Adams

"The Prayer"—Donnie McClurkin & Yolanda Adams

"He's Able"—Kirk Franklin

"Shackles (Praise You)"—Mary Mary

"Hello, Fear"—Kirk Franklin

"Change Me"—Tamela Man

"God Provides"—Tamela Mann

"I Got That"—Anthony Brown & group therAPy

"Won't He Do It"—Koryn Hawthorne

"Put a Praise on It"—Tasha Cobbs

"Smile"—Tasha Cobbs

"You Still Love Me"—Tasha Cobbs

"Confidence"—Tasha Cobbs

"Solid Rock"—Tasha Cobbs

"Cheers to the Fall"—Andra Day

"I Didn't Know My Own Strength"—Whitney Houston

"Greater Is Coming"—Jekalyn Carr

"Be Still"—Yolanda Adams

"Yes"—Shekinah Glory

"Jesus"—Shekinah Glory

"In His Presence"—Jekalyn Carr

"Already Won"—Jekalyn Carr

"The Hill"—Travis Green

"Reap"—J. J. Hairston & Youthful Praise

"Psalm 23 (I Am Not Alone)"—People and Songs

"Unstoppable"—Koryn Hawthorne

"Something Following Me"—Deon Kipping

"He Knows My Name"—Tasha Cobbs

"Symphony"—Switch

Review/Ask

L ove this book? Don't forget to leave a review! Every review matters, and it matters a *lot!* Head over to Amazon or wherever you purchased this book to leave an honest review for me. I thank you endlessly for taking the time to read this book. I pray it helped you in some way.

About the Author

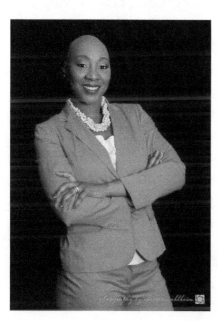

Anastasia R. Stevenson is a driven and respected leader known for executing on business strategy, developing teams, and driving results. She currently serves as director of project management at Cigna/Express Scripts. In this role, she is responsible for providing business direction and project management for strategic projects.

As a community advocate, Anastasia presently sits on the board of Mathews-Dickey Boys' and Girls' Club whose focus is to provide structured recreational activities to neighborhood youths. The club's goals are aimed at producing physically active, well-educated, and hopeful youth. Anastasia is also a strong community advocate for breast cancer, serving as an MBC ANGEL with the Tigerlily Foundation and ambassador on The Pink Angels Foundation.

Anastasia had the distinct pleasure of being recognized as one of the members of the Regional Business Council's Leadership 100, which is a network of up and coming young, diverse business professionals who pool their energy, enthusiasm, and skills to change the face of St. Louis. She has also been recognized as a leader in the workplace via the YWCA and Express Scripts and Professional Development Advocate of the Year by Mathews-Dickey Boys' and Girls' Club in 2018.

Anastasia obtained her bachelor of arts in human resource management from Webster University in Saint Louis, Missouri, and also earned her master of science in project management/information management in 2010 and, shortly after, completed her MBA in 2014 from Grantham University in Kansas City, Kansas. Anastasia is an avid learner and has completed the FOCUS St. Louis Emerging Leaders program and the St. Louis Business Diversity Initiative program.

Family is extremely important to Anastasia. She is happily in love with and married to *the* Prince Charming, Corey Stevenson Sr. (ten years), and they have three amazing children—Corey Jr. and twins Kennedi Neveah and Aaliyah Heaven. Together, they enjoy playing board games and spending lots of quality time together. Anastasia is also the youngest child to her mom, Eloise McClendon, and dad, Howard Gordon Sr.

CPSIA information can be obtained
at www.ICGtesting.com
Printed in the USA
BVHW082306060721
611232BV00008B/435